YES, YOU CAN

Dr. Harikrishna Devsare

DIAMOND BOOKS

Publisher	**:**	**Diamond Pocket Books (P) Ltd.**
		X-30, Okhla Industrial Area, Phase-II
		New Delhi-110020
Phone	:	011-40712200
E-mail	:	wecare@diamondbooks.in
Website	:	www.diamondbooks.in
Edition	:	2025
Printed by	:	Repro (India)

Yes, You Can

By : Harikrishan Devsare

Foreword

The importance of life lies in the fact that it is committed for an ambitious goal. Life is a theory of dynamism and not being static. Progressing continuously is the true meaning of life; it does not allow you to be static.

Jawahar Lal Nehru

Life is precious and is like a story. It is not important how long it is, but how beautiful it is.

Seneka – Roman visionary

We all live, but it is an open and debatable question as to who is really *successful* in life. Who lags behind in life? God made us one and gave life to one and all, but society created differences – caste, creed, religion, sex and so on – a difficult task indeed. Many great men, scientists, thinkers, saints and visionaries have tried to define success and life. This topic is quite complex and has been questioned throughout the ages. People have accepted this difference and experienced it in every era. This is a fact. A visionary said, 'Life is an unending festival for the indefatigable. They win by making efforts and bearing setbacks in life's battle.' There are complexities, problems and difficulties in life. We have to cross them to reach our destination. We can claim success by reaching our destination and find another goal at that point. We rejoice at the completion of our goals, and love to move ahead and achieve more. We have to climb hills of failure, cross oceans of difficulties and face the fire of discomforts. We hear only one voice - 'Win, if you can'. We have to move ahead with potential. Every step in our success is called a 'milestone' and we achieve it through sheer hard work, confidence, commitment and passion. Our self-confidence is the key to success and we need to nurture it. One can hope that this book will aid you. I can only say, 'Win, if you can'.

–Harikrishna Devsare

CONTENTS

1

WIN, IF YOU CAN

- *Your Victory*
- *Do it with passion*
- *Concentration is the formula for success*
- *Strong commitment has immense power*
- *Rock and human*
- *Faith in God*
- *Words of Intelligence*
- *Be away from 'Ifs' and 'Buts'*

Your victory

Life is like a game. We cannot control victory or defeat, but we can play.

It is true that defeat or victory lies in the game. We know that the result will be according to our performance. But our ego steps in and we follow it rather than trying to find the secret of playing well. We expect to win all the time. We think, 'Who can stop us?' The truth is that any egoist is sure to fail – and there are plenty of examples in every field. Big players have lost due to ego and have had to face defeat. Therefore, one has to beat the shortcomings obstructing one's path.

Orison Swett Marden said, 'One needs immense dedication to win.' Take the example of America's former president Roosevelt – if he had worked half-heartedly towards his goals, he would never have been so popular. He had only one secret of success in his life, i.e., he dedicated his life towards achieving his goals. He concentrated his energy on a single task and never shied away from doing it, and always completed what he started.

We all have some expectations from life and these make our life beautiful and simple. This is the basis of our success. You need to fix your goals before working on them. Someone said, 'Your goals must be most important in your life - they must be given top priority. It will enhance your energy, make you focused, and help you will move ahead. One who sets his targets firmly and makes sincere efforts to achieve them gains enormous power, and becomes creative and goal-oriented. But he needs to have a specific goal. He cannot succeed until he focuses his energy.'

If our mind is full of fear and doubts, we can't concentrate on our goal. Remove them, and you will find that you are able to balance your mind properly and work efficiently. One who concentrates, wins in life.

Whenever we do something, we hope to win and succeed. But it is necessary to let our self-confidence blossom and grow first. Great thinkers of the past have said, 'Work is not done by a person, but by his self-confidence. If there is any effective force in life which can enable one to succeed, it is self-confidence.' If you do a research on the successful people of this world, you will find self-confidence as their secret weapon of success. Man's energy and potential is only the source, but true force comes from confidence which makes us successful. Success is dependant upon capability, hard work and excellence in whatever we do. Some attribute success to their 'fate'. The truth is, it depends on the talent of the individual, and his capacity to recognize and avail of the opportunities that come his way.

You might have heard people say about a successful person that he is a 'Lucky Man.' But the truth is that the foundation of success lies in a healthy body and mind, the courage and the enthusiasm to follow one's goals through, and the ability to stay focussed. One who is ready to work hard, always wins. They have a dream and follow it dedicatedly – despite innumerable obstacles. No one can defeat a person of courage, hard-work, dedication and passion. His rivals eventually back off because he accomplishes his goals. History is full of people who have earned money and respect by overcoming poverty, social stigmas, etc. Their success was a result of their belief, confidence and hard work.

Then, there are people who try to use shortcuts in order to achieve success. They want instant success, but face failure at the end. The reason is their hurry to achieve their goals with minimum work. So, work with patience, believe in a good education, and move ahead in life.

Orison Swett Marden wrote, 'One needs to have consistency in his work to succeed, and not hurriedness.' When you will gain expertise in your field you will be appreciated by others, but working with hurriedness and impatience results in failure and embarrassment. Every dream requires a strong foundation, hard-work and research to make it come true. Every task requires patience and tolerance.

This is the secret to succeed and win in life. You will be with successful people who have never stopped moving forward in their lives. Naturally, they have won, and they have succeeded. You will win and succeed, too. Have confidence in yourself. As your confidence grows, your destination will become clearer and you will succeed. Have confidence, realize your true potential, be honest with yourself, and you will succeed.

Do it with passion

A person becomes impatient when surrounded by problems and difficulties. He needs to think about the solution, and needs to concentrate. This knowledge is gained from great men, thinkers and visionaries. Marcus Aurelius, the Roman emperor, was a great thinker and visionary. He used to discuss his problems out loud with himself and find solutions to them. It has influenced and inspired many lives. 'The world is 'living', and you are part of it. It's our natural instincts to benefit the world through our thoughts and deeds. You have to think intelligibly to benefit yourself.'

Marcus wrote, 'Everything happens for a reason. Parent DNA's come together, and that is the reason for a new life. Every thing in this world is under God's control. Not even an atom can work against it. You are a part of it. Never feel depressed about any incident in your life. Everything changes with time. This is nature's rule, and you should find peace by being aware of this truth. Proceed in your life with this rule.'

The purpose of human life is to achieve something meaningful and useful, and in accomplishing our goals. Marcus said, 'You have spent your days without setting goals, you have wasted much time. So don't delay anymore. Discover the truth and find a peaceful state. What is this world all about? Who is the governor of this universe? You are the spark of the fire of the universe. Your time is precious. So, let the light of knowledge enter your mind and ward off the darkness in your heart. Follow your plans without worry or confusion, and follow them with passion. You might not get a second chance. Remove ego, dissatisfaction and jealousy from your mind.'

We are always caught between tension and peace. When we are happy, we fear failure. When we are unhappy, we are waiting for our happiness and remain worried. According to Marcus, we have trapped ourselves in this cycle. God has no role to play in it, so He should not be blamed. He explained, 'Both good and bad people have to face hardship. One cannot be partial about it.' God never created miseries or happiness in our lives. All is under His control - respect, insult, peace, difficulty – it does not happen according to the wishes of people. These things are not 'real'. We only have illusions of peace, and get attracted to it. We hesitate to face our problems. Some of us feed our egos till they become big and begin to rule us. This is useless and cannot benefit us. So, never get attracted to worthless articles. Know your inner self and accept it. Understand what is best for your soul.

According to Marcus, one will succeed in every task if his heart is pure. All we need is to concentrate and make a sincere effort. People who do crack the toughest examinations. Marcus goes on to write, 'Watch carpenters and artistes... they forget everything else when they are at work. You will find persistence in detail and exquisiteness of their art and their craft. They concentrate on their work, work with passion (sometimes even forgetting to sleep!), and give their best everytime. Naturally, they end up successful. Why aren't *you* performing *your* best for *your* success?'

Marcus said 'Whatever you do, do it with passion, intelligence and persistence. Never think about useless things. Never interfere with others. Never hide your weakness. Think of God who created you and be a king of your dreams. Be happy and peaceful.'

Concentration is the formula for success

This is not a story of mountaineers but a story of success and failure that continues to inspire us. It says clearly: *Despite setbacks, you will succeed in the end.* This is about team spirit. I was reading about a research on the famous Mount Everest conquest in 1963. Norman Dinferth was the leader of the group, while Jim and Sherpa Twang Gombu were his teammates. They were climbing the steepest slope. It was 28,400 feet above sea level, and they had emptied half of their oxygen bottles in order to reduce their weight (thinking that the oxygen they had will be sufficient for the rest of their journey). They reached the peak at 11:30, but got caught in a heavy storm. Confused, they didn't know whether to go or stop. Jim thought it was a steep slope ahead, and that it would be difficult to proceed. Soon, they were 30 feet within summit distance, and continued to climb carefully. They reached Hilary's chimney on the side of Kanchanjunga, and started observing the place. From where he stood, Jim could see the mountain peak jutting magnificently into the sky. He said to Gombu, 'Gombu, you move first,'. But Gombu was not tall, and asked Jim to proceed. So, Jim said 'Let's walk together.' They began to move ahead with each other's support. It was 1 pm, and they had traveled for 7 hours, when they finally reached the top. Jim jabbed a 4 feet aluminum stick into the summit surface, and tied his country's flag to it.

This is a great example of team work, courage, humanity and persistence. Jim could have reached Everest first, but he waited for Gombu and decided to reach there together. In life, we have to learn to walk with others.

The expedition to Mount Everest has always been the symbol of courage and self- confidence. Over generations, mountaineers who have scaled its peak (and refused to give up) have provided us valuable lessons in determination and fortitude. Whatever life demands of you, whatever the challenges, we have to make a solid effort and move on ahead. Our passion for our work will make the journey easier. Passion is the spark that has the difficultly to destroy all our difficulties. All we need is to focus. Khalil Gibran said, 'Put all your physical and mental energies into your goals in life, and you will succeed.'

A famous thinker once said, 'Energy and concentration is your victory, which brings about miraculous transformations in your life.' Those who have conquered the highest mountains, crossed the infinite skies and plumbed the deepest oceans for pearls inspire us with their stories of courage, and make us believe that we can also win by sheer effort and concentration. Marle wrote, 'One has to be focused in order to gain victory in any task in life. Those who work in different directions never taste success.'

A thinker once said, 'All those who arose and shone amongst their peers did so by dint of their commitment and capabilities. They were otherwise common men and women, like everyone else.' Victor Hugo said, 'We don't lack potential, but dedication.' One needs dedication and commitment for any task to be completed. One can conquer defeat with these qualities. They enlighten and energize us, and help us fend off disgrace and difficulties in our journey towards success. Julius Caesar became a legend with the help of his dynamism, dedication and commitment.

Strong commitment has immense power

One day Lord Buddha was travelling with his followers, when they came upon a giant stone on the road. One of them asked 'Lord, can anyone be stronger than this?'

The Lord said, 'Yes, iron is stronger than stone. It can break it into pieces.'

The follower asked, 'Is there anything stronger than iron?'

Buddha replied, 'Yes, fire. It can melt iron and make it soft like liquid.'

The follower asked, 'Nobody can conquer fire.'

Buddha replied, 'That's not true. Water can easily extinguish fire.'

'Who can dare challenge the power of water? It can create floods.'

Buddha said, 'Wind can change the course of water. Air is also vital for life on earth.'

The follower asked, 'So which is the thing, or the force, that is stronger than even wind?'

Buddha replied, 'The strongest of all is commitment, which can conquer air. It is the strongest power in this universe.'

Commitment is definitely the strongest force, and is the formula for success in any field. The one who shows commitment with passion succeeds in life. All great men have used this tool to achieve their goals.

A thinker has written 'Commitment has a strange power. An inspired person can move ahead with commitment and passion. It automatically blocks all exit-ways of going back, and destroys all obstructions on the way.' Abraham Lincoln wrote about American Independence in his diary, 'I have committed to complete this task in front of God.' This gave him the capability to achieve his goal. All our senses start working with commitment and concentration. Candy , the eminent thinker, said, 'When a desire for something grows strongly inside you, you start believing that God has safeguarded it for you. Your commitment and belief get stronger, and you inevitably succeed.'

You have to decide your goal, your target. You cannot move a step without it. In fact, there is no meaning or use of life without purpose. It is like a boat sailing without direction. If you have any goal, work towards it. Just thinking about it won't make you successful. You have to stay alert and motivated all the time. Actor Wilfton Kapde was criticized when he began acting. But he was committed to his passion, and improved his acting skills steadily, day and day. Eventually, he became a famous and successful star. His secret? Focusing all his energies into every single task. Until a person applies all his energy in his work, he will never succeed.

One needs a well-focused mind for success. Great people concentrated on their dreams, and did not waste their energy on useless tasks. Swett Marden wrote 'Hesitation is a sign of weakness. A person fails due to two reasons – lack of commitment for his plan and doubts about it.' The secret of success is being dedicated towards your goal during the hardest and darkest of times, and finding inspirations and solutions from it.

Rock and human

We generally think about completing our tasks, but fail to prioritize them. As a result, we cannot start any job, and even when we do so, we can't finish it. This happens during important times like exams, competitions and official projects. When time is less, we do what we can, but do not get the desired results (we jumble things up). We alone are responsible for it, but instead, we blame others. If we analyze deeply, we will realize the real causes of failure – Our lack of dedication and passion. It's important to realize the importance of commitment in life.

It's an old story – you might have read it. There was a village. When it rained, it didn't reach the village; Instead, it rained on the other side of the mountain. Everyone said that the mountain was stopping the rain. So what could be done? One angry farmer decided to raze it to the ground, and started digging. The mountain saw the man's commitment, and prayed to God. When Lord Vishnu appeared, the mountain said, 'Lord, look... the farmer is trying to destroy me because he thinks I stop the rain.' The Lord said, 'Why are you scared? He alone cannot do anything.' The mountain replied, 'I am scared of his commitment. If he cannot do it alone, his friends and sons will surely get the job done. Please save me.' Lord said, 'If he is so committed then I cannot do anything. One who has dedication can never fail in his life. So, you will have to wait and see the result of his dedication.'

Emerson, the eminent thinker, once said, 'History is witness to the defeat of evil, demons and inequity against human dedication.'

Helen Keller said, 'The one who acts with courage and dedication not only achieves his or her goals, but assures others of success as well.' When I was a sophomore, I wrote "I believe in God, humanity and potential of each individual... I consider it my duty to be courageous, and inspire others similarly. I should not criticize the creation of God. In fact, no one has the right to speak against nature because God has created it beautifully, and we all need to preserve it." A long time has passed, and I have bore many shocks, but have never felt the need to change nature. One who believes God is an optimist. He knows that truth will prevail in the end... and that he (or she) is always surrounded by God's support.'

Commitment is the foundation of success. In life, we are faced with fears and problems. But if they cause us to deviate from our path, we cannot achieve our goals. So, we should remain dedicated. Gandhiji said, 'Commitment is like a place which protects us from temptation and keeps us still.'

We need emotional and mental stability more than physical strength to achieve success. If we have no commitment, then we cannot accomplish our goal even with great physical resources. So it is said that 'One needs less of money and more of heart to do good for others.'

Commit and complete. When a person becomes dedicated, he becomes dynamic and starts believing in his inner super power. Such a person is sure to succeed.

Faith in God

There was once a man who was addicted to smoking and drinking. His addictions made him depressed, but he couldn't do anything about it. One day, he read in a book, 'Commitment has immense power... practice it, and watch the miracles that follow.' He thought about it, and decided to try it. No matter how tempted he was, he never touched cigarettes or alcohol again. He stuck to his resolve, and succeeded. Encouraged, he decided to practice the same in other situations of life. He succeeded everywhere. He became an inspiration for others, and was like a brand new person! How could people refuse to believe that dedication has a strong power inside?

Commitment is a formula that can help you to succeed in any area of life. Doctors, engineers, scientists and psychologists have acknowledged the power of commitment, and experienced the miracles. One doctor writes 'Commitment has great power which can enable even a handicap to get up and run. We can call it energy, which not only cures you but also protects you from other diseases.' We can generate positive energy through our commitment, and it can support us at every step to think positively and gain in confidence. It helps us fight daily challenges with ease.

One person explained inner potential simply as will-power. When you decide to do something, you commit yourself to it, and, instantly, a burning desire is generated. Just as current flows through an electronics gadget the moment the switch is turned on, similarly, our will-power fills us instantly with positive energy. One who has this energy can apply it in any dimension, to achieve anything. We meet people who are energetic and bring charm in everything they say or do. On the other hand, there are those who can demoralize even others with their own lethargy. So, if you want to increase your will-power and become energetic, then meet those who have an abundance of it. They can transmit their force to you, and make you self-confident.'

Many people have succeeded in this world because of commitment. When they decided to succeed, they worked with passion, energy and perseverance to win. Their success stories inspired others to be like them. It was their commitment that made them fight difficulties. Marco Polo completed his journey to China, Russia, Burma, Java, Sumatra and Sri Lanka. Columbus discovered the West Indies and America: His chronicles describes in detail the obstacles he faced along his journey, and the way he overcame them. Vasco De Gama found the passage to India, and opened new avenues for trade for the world. James Crook found East Australia, New Zealand and Antarctica, followed by the Hawaii Islands and the Sahara desert. He was a man fiercely committed to his dreams. There are many examples of commitment and dedication that have altered the course of history, and changed our lives forever.

There are many people in this world who have accomplished their task by risking their lives on the principle of commitment. They are people who were committed, and finished every task they began. They repeated the rules of success in their minds and moved on the path of success – stopping after every triumph to gather energy for the next challenge. Their decision never changed, and they steadily gained in confidence. The more the confidence, the more the success. If you have to wake up early in the morning, say to yourself, 'I'll get up at 4 am in the morning.' Go to sleep with this commitment and you *will* wake up at that time. Gandhiji said, 'Commitment guards us against temptations, and protects us from being weak and feeble.' So, the basic requirement for success is commitment. Try to apply it in your life, and you will find amazing results. Someone rightly said, 'Strong commitment is the true worship of God.'

Words of intelligence

'If there is any intelligent thought, it is concentration: A foolish act scatters your thoughts. Concentration flushes out all illusions from our minds and enables us to work from our heart.'

We fail to do even simple tasks when we lack commitment. Our energy is scattered – this is a scientific truth. If that energy is focused at one point, then it becomes easier to reach our goal. If you have played a game of burning cotton with a convex lens or magnifying glass, you know how powerful concentrated energy can be. 'Concentration is your secret power to win. It foregathers all the faculties and potential of a person to succeed in life.' In our routine life, our mind usually lies scattered in several different things. We have to concentrate before every task we undertake. When we are busy, we say 'Just a minute: I'm thinking about something!' The reason is that our 'inner mind' cannot focus on too many tasks at once. One should know how to prioritize things, and focus on a single item at a time. Someone who has learnt this 'trick', is the king of his mental powers.

When we talk of concentration, it means putting all our energy in the goals to be achieved – be it an exam to be cleared, or an important job interview. If we chase two rabbits, both will escape. One never succeeds while preparing for two competitions simultaneously. People who multi-task seldom succeed in life. It is said that one cannot sail in two boats. But people still try to. There is a saying 'Concentration is the pre-condition for one's success. If our energy is scattered, success becomes unattainable.' Orison Swett Marden said, 'One person has only one main quality. If he applies his potential with that quality, he can succeed. But having 10 qualities and no concentration is a sure way to fail. Even the weakest person can achieve his goals by focusing on them.'

Concentration is the power that works like a magnet and attracts success to it. Abraham Lincoln is well known for his art of focusing. Victor Hugo closed his room until he completed his writing. Orison Swett Marden writes, 'If a person hesitates to do something, it is his weakness. There are two reasons of failure – Lack of decision, and doubts before any task. He cannot focus due to these and thus remains unsuccessful.' Johann Wolfgang von Goethe said, 'Be there, wherever you are. Do it once, and do it best. Concentrate all your energy in the task you are going to perform well. Don't worry about the results. Never regret after doing your job.'

In spirituality, concentration means meditation. If the mind is wandering, then it cannot concentrate and one cannot succeed whether he is working on a machine, appearing for exam or doing anything else. McDougall wrote in 'Outline of Psychology', the mind has to play an important role in meditating, to concentrate on a particular task. We cannot work without concentration.' Woodworth said, 'Our mind reacts to some selected actions from a set of uncountable actions every moment. It concentrates on one or a set of tasks at a time.' Concentration means to be alert and dynamic towards a particular event. If you focus on something, you eliminate other useless thoughts. Sidney Smith said that forgetting irrelevant and unimportant events is the real meaning of concentration. Meredith explained that one who looks for only one thing he believes in, will get it before he dies. Orison Swett Marden also says that no task can remain incomplete, if done with concentration.

Be away from 'Ifs' and 'Buts'

This is a story of Subhash Chandra Bose and his commitment. A fatal, hazardous disease had spread in a village called Jaajpur. Subhash wanted to help the patients. His Guru Benimadhav tried to stop him, but could not influence him. He knew that Subhash would do it if he was committed to it. Therefore, he allowed him to go to Jaajpur and also went with him. The two served there for two months and then came back. Subhash's father asked, 'Where were you for such a long time?' Subhash replied, 'I was in Jaajpur'. His father was shocked and said, 'Why did you go there?' Subhash replied, 'To help the patients.' His father asked him about his knowledge of the disease. He replied, 'Just like you worry about me, I think about others. People were dying without treatment. So it was my duty to serve them.' His father roared, 'Son of Rai Bahadur Jankidas Bose, who has enough servants in his house, went to serve others? Didn't you think about my status? You forgot that you are the child of a Rai Bahadur who is respected by officers.' Subhash said, 'I don't think I have insulted you in any manner. In fact, I have made you respectable by saving others' lives. People were praising you for giving me birth.' His father was left speechless.

When we commit ourselves to a decision, we leave no scope for any 'ifs' and 'buts'. All we need to do is believe that, 'Yes, I can', and work to reach our goals. No one can stop us from succeeding. Any circumstance can be dealt with and overcome with commitment. For such people, the whole world makes way for success.

Confucius said, 'You cannot defeat anyone's commitment, even if you defeat his soldiers.'

There are many examples of great people with towering commitment. American president Abraham Lincoln, the French Emperor Napoleon, Roman king Julius Caeser – their lives inspire us even today.

'One who is always ready to work hard with his sleeves rolled up never exhausts from his work, and never shies from working in dust, storm or any other adversity. The youth should learn to become great by challenging fate and triumphing over their destiny.'

❑

2

PRAYER & SPIRITUALITY

- *Why should we pray?*
- *Be Polite*
- *Grow your will-power*
- *Prayer does not make you fortunate*
- *Importance of patience*
- *Be away from jealousy*
- *Key to Success*
- *Desires will be accomplished*
- *Faith and duty*
- *Science and spirituality are inter-related to each other*

Why should we pray?

We pray to God before initiating any task. Why do we pray? We pray because we believe ourselves to be feeble in comparison to God. A social thinker once wrote, 'The meaning of prayer is to make us believe that we should get rewards as per our capabilities and as we deserve. It is to keep our soul happy. This is self-acknowledgement. If the mind is controlled, everything can be under control. If one becomes capable, then why would he need to sit among losers and cry for their fate and ask destiny's help?'

When we pray with a pure heart, that is the truest prayer. When people shout on mikes and ring large bells, is it a real prayer? Is the focus truly on God when they do so? If not, then why do we expect results from it? A true prayer is one in which we concentrate. A saying goes, 'We link ourselves to the almighty cosmic force through prayer and gain the confidence of strong relations with Him. God is witness, creator, governor, director, executor and everything else, but we should pray to the pure part of God. Only the inner glow of satisfaction and success is asked through the prayer.'

Some people say that prayer is not useful. I have prayed to God everyday but never benefited. You will find some people saying, 'God helped me, so I always visit the temple on tuesdays.' Many temples have idols of Shiva, Hanuman or Ganesha - deities known for fulfilling desires. For the same reason, people visit Vaishno Devi, Siddhi Vinayak, Haji Ali and Khwaja. A thinker has tried to elaborate it by saying, 'Prayer is heard when made with a pure heart. The heart is aware of all the things and wants to get more, but merely asking is not enough. One has to make efforts to get something. It does not matter who you are - a beggar or a thief. If the thief steals from the temple, he will remain a thief. No amount of praying can make a difference to his life.'

One should not forget the importance of hard work, alongwith prayer. If we do not study and keep playing and roaming around, then praying just before the exams will not help us. Don't just blame God: One has to make the effort as well.

True prayer is one in which we ask God to give us knowledge. True prayer is one in which we ask God to give us the energy to gain victory, and not the victory itself. People might remember this prayer: 'Give us the power, so that we remain on the right path. We may succeed by serving others. Keep us away from fraud, fake and bogus ideas. Make our life pure and simple.'

A thinker has said, 'Prayer is sacrificing the ego and poor thoughts, in order to gain a better character.' So pray before starting any task, it will increase your confidence. This helps us increase our efforts, and we reach our destination. The process supports us throughout by inspirations along the way.

Be Polite

One can drink water under a waterfall only by bowing under it. This is a sign of politeness. It is an important part of our life. Those who are high thinkers are always polite. After achieving a certain amount of success in life, people tend to have inflated egos. They feel superior to others. Once the success has ended, they suddenly face defeat and humiliation for becoming one of the 'inferiors' again. Therefore, one should sacrifice ego and be polite.

The third Sikh Guru, Guru Amar Das, strengthened the practice of Langar (free kitchen), which was started by Guru Nanak. It was the injunction of **Guru Amar Das** that none would have his audience unless he had first eaten from the Langar. The Guru intended to remove the caste restrictions and prejudices of untouchability. It was, therefore, declared unequivocally that all persons of all castes, high or low, rich or poor, Brahmans or Shudras, Hindus or Muslims, must sit in the same line and eat the same food from Guru's kitchen. The idea was to bring the different communities together. His message spread widely. Akbar, the Mughal emperor, was a religious person. He too appreciated the idea and decided to meet the Guru. He sent a message that he wanted to meet Amar Das and Amar Das agreed to meet him – but he said that all were equal here, and so Akbar would have to participate in the Langar. Akbar agreed. Amar Das said, 'One can be a follower if he has trust, discipline and politeness in his heart.'

In reality, the more a person is polite the greater he becomes. Ego cannot touch him. They don't cry on their fate nor blame others for their failure. They are peaceful and find constructive solutions to their problems.

Some people feel disappointed and discouraged after failing just once. This is wrong. It is natural to make mistakes in life, and one should learn from them and try not to repeat it. It is possible if you do not have any ego, and we are polite and peaceful. These people are optimists and creative, they have the capacity to accomplish a task. They don't have any ego. They are always polite. The egoist people only find faults in others and qualities in themselves. They never appreciate others and remain worried in life. A thinker said, 'I have seen people succeeding only when they are happy and optimist. They set their goals before initiating any task. They never show egotism in their behavior but have confidence. Then one who boasts of his potential doesn't know it well. He is not aware of the extremities and shortcomings. He suffers from a wrong verdict and fails in life.' Those who know their potential decide their goals beforehand so that they may use it to their greatest advantage. Ego detours us from our path. There are many holy books explaining the consequences of ego. Ravana and Kans were defeated because of their ego. It is good to adopt politeness in life. One who does so is always gentle to others, never boasts of his qualities and is respected everywhere.

This is an old story. The lid of a pot had a huge ego because it kept the water pure all the time and it was sitting on the topmost place. It once asked the pot, 'You supply water to others and keep me thirsty. Don't you know my importance?' The pot replied, 'It is not my fault – you are sitting on my head. If you come down, I can supply you the water.' The lid, of course, remains thirsty to this day! It is clear that an egotist never reaches his destination. So sacrifice it and move ahead in life.

Grow your will power

Osho (Bhagwan Shree Rajneesh) says, 'People come to me and complain of not finding peace, inability to meditate, etc. I tell them to stop worrying about peace. Only meditate and you will find it. They return after 15 days and repeat the same. Many people become spiritual because of greed and expect heaven and its conveniences. But they do not know the real place of it. Your heaven is not waiting for you. Likewise, there is no hell as such. This is imaginary. A person asked his servant in Arab to light a fire for smoking. His servant found fire at different places but could not bring it. Then the master said 'Bring it from hell' and the servant reached there. The gatekeeper said, 'Go inside and take it' but he could not find fire and came out and asked the gatekeeper, 'I had heard of fire inside but could not find it here. Where should I get it from?' The gatekeeper said, 'Every person brings his own fire with him. Hell and heaven are inside. It is not in your future but in your present. It is all about your attitude, you can create heaven or hell as you wish. There are people who find heaven in hell because their heaven lies inside. As of now, you are trying to be religious for peace but you are unable to do so as it is inside you. You need to identify it.'

Actually peace and anxiety, hope and despair, success and failure, all lie inside us. We need to identify them because only then can we discover our inner potential. Thinkers and visionaries have stated that our inner potential shapes our character. But our ego stops us from this path of self-discovery. We are engulfed in vanity; we are obsessed with our self. We think we can answer the toughest questions, yet the simplest ones always baffle us. We make obvious mistakes, but lie under the illusion that we knew the answer and wrote it well. Naturally, when we fail, we tend to blame others for it. We forget that we didn't use our inner potential while answering the questions because we were filled with ego. We have to blame ourselves, nobody else. Hence, we have to identify our strengths and weaknesses and work towards improving our character. Only then can we grow our will power, which will inspire us in every walk of life.

French poet Victor Hugo said, 'We do not lack energy but will-power. One needs commitment and dedication to complete a great job. One can cross all the barriers by self-acknowledgement and self-awareness. We need to feel the spark of will-power in his body. Only then can we proceed forward with improvement and improvisation, tackling circumstances, growing hope. All great people rose amongst their contemporaries by will-power and realizing their inner potential. They were 'common men and women' just like others in all other aspects.'

Prayer does not make you fortunate

One doesn't become fortunate by praying. If such had been the case, then only the devout religious people and fanatics would have achieved success. That would have reduced the importance of prayer as well. Those who think that they can escape from work by praying are wrong. Prayer cannot take the place of work, and vice-versa. If it had been so, then a doctor would have prayed to God instead of operating on his patient. Prayer makes us polite and civil, which is essential to life. It helps us practise our powers of concentration. The importance of concentration has already been explained to you. Prayer is not begging in front of God.

It means to empower yourself to succeed, to accept the challenges and win. Concentration is gained through prayer. And through concentration towards our goal, we gain success. We cannot attribute this success to fortune – it is sheer hard work paying off.

Here's another story. The founder of the Ghaznavid empire, emperor Mahmud-e-Ghaznawi, had appointed a shepherd, Ayaz, as his bishop after he came to know about his intelligence. The boy continuously impressed the emperor. His companions were envious of him. Ayaz had cited one condition – he would not work between 8 to 9 am – and Ghaznawi accepted it. One day, a show piece was stolen and everyone blamed Ayaz. They went to his house in search of the show piece and knocked on the door. Ayaz reminded them about the condition, but his mates persuaded him to open the door. He finally opened the door, but they could not find anything in his house. They noticed Ayaz holding a bag tightly. They urged him to open the bag and Ayaz refused to do so. At last, the bag was opened and they saw old clothes used by Ayaz to graze his sheep. There was a cap and a stick. Mahmud Ghaznawi asked about it. Ayaz replied, 'You appointed me to the high post of a bishop but I do not want to forget my old roots... that I am a shepherd. So I see myself in the mirror every day, so that I do not forget my old days. I pray to God to protect me from becoming an egotist, and to help me walk the path of honesty.' Ghaznawi was extremely glad to hear this. He punished the people who had blamed the shepherd, and, later, promoted Ayaz to kingship. So was this an act of fortune, or was it the result of honesty, intelligence, hardwork and loyalty of Ayaz?

Vinobha Bhave said, 'Prayer blesses us with power. Asking for the correct utilization of this power is the true meaning of prayer.' When we pray to God, Allah or Ishwar, we are asking for the power to work, and not directly demanding for success. Fortune is achieved in this way. There are no short-cuts to it.

Mahatma Gandhi said, 'Prayer is an abbreviation of religion. It is not demanding, but humbly asking, for a pure mind and soul. It is the acceptance of our weaknesses, and the internal process by which we 'evaluate' and 'correct' ourselves.' Gandhiji used to pray every day but not for independence. He always asked for energy to fight with the British, and he ended up achieved his goal! Gandhiji explained the meaning of prayer as 'It is the sense of purity that promotes and begets politeness, and gives us the energy to partner our fellow men in their times of trouble and adversity.'

This means that prayer doesn't make one fortunate instantly like magic, but helps us face the right direction in life. Gandhiji was never 'fortunate He had to work hard for every little thing he got in life. He never worried about the results, he kept on working towards his goals. True Prayer doesn't teach us to be a blind follower. Those who shirk work never reap the results of prayer. Prayer is not to make you an escapist, but to give you the energy and focus to work harder.

Prayer and success are two completely separate things. Prayer never makes you clear the exams without studying. Only an idle mind can think of such a thing. If peace, politeness and tolerance are man's ornaments, then their roots lie in the prayer. If compulsivity, passion and hard work are essential for human life, then these are the ingredients of success as well. Both prayer and success are important, and have their own value and place. You have to choose them according to your need. As physical growth requires many ingredients, success cannot be attained with a single quality. We have to grasp the best to be successful – this is the formula.

Importance of patience

One day, Lord Buddha was travelling with his follower Mahakashyap. Mahakashyap used to ask many questions from the Lord to find solutions. He asked, 'Lord, the soul is internal, untouchable and unmanageable. How can we stabilize it? It is very difficult to control both mind and soul. How can we purify our soul?' Lord Buddha did not reply instantly. He did not want to dishearten his follower, but he wanted to wait for the right time to answer the questions. One day while taking rest under a tree in scorching heat, he asked his follower to bring water to drink. Mahakashyap went but returned without water. He said that an animal had polluted the water, so he would have to bring water from the river. Buddha replied that the river was quite far, so he must go to the waterfall for pure water. Mahakashyap went there, and brought clean water. Buddha drank the water and said, 'You had asked a question from me. The answer is that you have to keep your heart patient, just like this water. Water is clean at its source but becomes dirty on roaming around; So does the heart.'

If we do our job patiently, we can succeed. If we hurry and want instant results, then we will only face disappointment and losses. If Mahakashyap had brought the dirty water from the nearby place, it could have made them ill. Similarly, hurried actions do not bring good results. Our heart forces us to work faster. If we have studied hard, and know the answers, but write them hurriedly, the results will not be as good as we expect them to be. And then we blame others for no reason, without acknowledging the real cause.

Patience examines our nature and character closely. Sant Kabir said, *'Kabira dhiraj ke dhare, haathi man bhar khaye; took ek ke karne, swan ghare ghar jaaye.'* The one who is patient and never wanders or expects results, surely succeeds in life. John Ruskin has written, 'Patience is the root of all powers and peace.'

The great philosopher Ralph Waldo Emerson said, 'Analyze nature, and you'll see that its secret is patience.' There is no better teacher than nature. Everything happens with time and patience. The seeds that we sow will reap at the right time, and we have to wait for the rain and harvesting time. As nature works patiently with time, we also need to learn from it. French visionary Jean Jacques Rousseau said, 'Patience is bitter, but its result is sweet.'

Kabir wrote, *'Dheere dheere re mana, dheere sub kuchh hoyae, maali seenche sau garha, ritu aaye fal hoye.'* We get many opportunities in life, but we have to work patiently. There is no other option. One can cure and rectify himself only by patience. The doctor gives medicine to his patients, and the medicine cures on time – not later, nor earlier; We have to wait for the right moment for everything in life. Rishi Valmiki said, 'One who exercises patience in hard times and financial crisis, and uses his brain, never feels sad.'

Whenever we come across any challenge, we have to keep patience. In other words, we have to stabilize our confidence. Whatever the circumstance, we should not lose our confidence. This will take us to great heights.

Be away from jealousy

We know the story about Mahmud Ghaznawi and Ayaz (chapter 'Prayer does not make you fortunate'). His mates were envious of him because of the important position he held in Mahmud Ghaznawi's court. They were continuously trying to find faults in Ayaz. Mahmud Ghaznavi understood their nature and was fed up of their complaints. So he decided to teach them a lesson. One day, a troop came to the city. The Emperor was sitting in his court. The sheriff ordered one of his men to go and find out where they are coming from. The man returned and said that they had come from Bagdad. The

Emperor wanted to know where they were headed. Again, a man was sent and came back to say that they were on their way to Damishk. Emperor asked about the number of people and asked a third person to gather this information. He returned and told the Emperor that there were 50 people. Then, Gazni wanted to know the purpose of their arrival. The next person was quiet. But Ayaz came later and said, 'They have come from Bagdad and are on their way to Damishk. There are 25 camels, 20 males, 20 females and 10 kids. They are here to trade for wheat, pulses, etc. Ibrahim, a veteran and believer of God, is the leader of this group.' The emperor turned to his sheriff and said, 'Did all of you hear Ayaz? He gathered as much information as he could at one go, on his own. Those who envy him should learn from him. A jealous person never has the solution... in fact, he is the problem.'

Jealousy is a bad habit. It is present in every place, era and age. Kids feel jealous because of lack of toys while a student envies a brilliant student. People envy their successful neighbours, players, etc. Offices and businesses are other places where we see rampant jealousy. Someone rightly said, 'Jealousy is a small trap which can create disaster in our lives. It pitches your life dangerously up and down at every moment. Those who know it play safe, and remain stable and calm always.'

Why do we become jealous? It is because we do not become what we want to be. Human wants are unlimited, and we are never satisfied. An 'illusion of failure' (if you analyse deeply, you will find that each of us are successful in some way or the other!) causes jealousy, and, as a result, we start criticizing others instead of appreciating them and their success. Would we be successful even if the other person was not? No. Jealousy provokes the wrong thoughts in our minds about others... and we never try to analyse the real reasons of our failure.

A jealous person forgets that he is putting himself in trouble. We are always busy in finding others' weaknesses, and easily forget our own shortcomings. As a result, we do not grow in life and remain envious of others' successes. We try to hurt them instead of concentrating on our strengths and weaknesses, and get hurt in the process. This negative mindset prevents us from being dynamic. We become lazy and unsuccessful. Someone has rightly said, 'A jealous person is always full of anxiety and surrounded by trouble. He always speaks badly of others and feels depressed by his neighbour's success.'

Hence, we should destroy the green-eyed monster called jealousy, and discover routes to improving our own inadequacies and shortcomings. This can be achieved by analyzing the reasons for others' success with an unhurried and clean mind, and by adopting them ourselves. A well known Hindi playwright, Jainendra Kumar, has said, 'Jealousy grows from dejection, and it only suppresses and worsens it.'

So, we should find our weaknesses rather than envying others. We should grow our confidence and adopt others' qualities to the best possible extent. We need to attain genuine values and principles of life. This will make us successful.

Key to success

Story time! There was a boy who decided to be rich, for he thought money would bring him peace and all happiness. He started his quest. First, he met a bully person. He was impressed with him and decided to become like him. He studied his nature. Then, halfway through, he met a musician and decided to be like him. One fine day, he met a saint and wanted to be like him. As a result, he could gain nothing in life. He grew old, and was neither a bully, a musician, a saint, or rich. He felt very depressed and discussed his feelings to a saint. The saint replied, 'This world is very attractive. We have many desires but everything cannot be attained in one go. So decide your goals and dedicate your life to it. Until you have commitment, you cannot succeed.'

Wishes are a part of our life. If there were no desires, our lives would become stagnant and meaningless. Desires, dreams and wishes inspire us to climb higher, and achieve great things in life. But then, human desires are endless. We want good food, clothes, luxuries, etc. Wishes only increase with time, and sometimes, we fail to fulfill them. Family, home, society, etc., are the results of wishes. Whatever we think we need, we desire. It means we want to shape our life according to our desires. But it is not possible to fulfill one's all wishes. Although it is not possible to stop these wishes from arising in our minds, they can certainly be controlled.

We dream but forget that we might not be capable of achieving it. Our success and failure depend on this crucial understanding. Those who do not realize it never identify their potential. A thinker said, 'Our emotions are like our desires, and can be clearly seen in our expressions.' It is necessary to control our desires because they affect our character. If these are not controlled, they may drive us to acts of extreme consequences, even crime. But if you control your desires, then it can be a stepping stone for you. A thinker once said, 'You must first dedicate yourself before starting a job so as to succeed in it.' If you want to succeed in any tough competition, then you will have to show your commitment. It takes enormous focus and energy in us to reach our goal. But our desire should be in accordance with our capacity so that our job becomes easy and our goals stay realistic. This will enable us to fight every obstacle with enthusiasm, and no one can stop us from succeeding. No one who lacks commitment has achieved success. Benjamin Disraeli, British

Statesman and literary figure, said, 'Man is not a slave of circumstances, but circumstances are the slaves of man.'

The world is full of thoughts. There is no wish that cannot be fulfilled. Jesus' life tells us to listen to our heart. You may have to sacrifice a few things to succeed in life, but be dedicated to your dreams and work patiently. People will criticize you and create obstacles in your way. They may call you mad, but you have to stay focused and move forward regardless. You have to carry your belief and commitment with you everywhere, and it will take you towards success. It will fill enormous confidence in you.

Orison Swett Marden said, 'If our will-power is weak, then our mind will work equally feebly, and will fail to support you.' Disraeli said, 'Your senses get attracted to what you desire and allure you towards it. Wishes are like seeds of success. Till the seed is sown, one cannot expect results. So, one cannot fulfill his desires without hard work and efforts. You may be surrounded by difficulties, but you should not lose confidence. Be patient, work hard, and reach your destination. Your confidence will get rid of all your obstacles.'

Desires will be accomplished

I was reading about Peter A Foster and how one can achieve the best qualities by paying their price. He wrote, 'It is said that the best things in life are free. These are things we value the most, like affection, peace, charm, etc. These do not come with a price tag. It doesn't, of course, mean they are totally free.'

Whatever is worth acquiring, has some price attached to it, but most people want to get it free. One who doesn't think of others' troubles can never discover true love. One cannot gain mental peace, charm and success without paying something in return. Making genuine efforts towards attaining a goal, maintaining them, and being optimist and patient are the chief reasons behind success. You have to pay for it, in the form of work or efforts. If you are ready to pay the price in the form of hard work, you will get the best results and you will succeed. The best things of life may be 'free', but one must still pay, by hard work.

Ibn Batuta, famous Moroccan scholar, emphasized the importance of hard work. 'A farmer has to work very hard in his field. Do the flowers grow by themselves? Only the person who has worked on them knows the patience and effort that have been invested behind it. Never forget to work hard. Each of your desire will be fulfilled because you have paid for it.'

It is a general phenomenon that people never accept the truth. They waste their efforts by escaping from the job, because their interest isn't in it. Working towards a purpose and desiring other goals simultaneously is a serious mistake. This sidetracks us from our main goal. As a result, we do not combine the power of sheer hard work, confidence and patience. One cannot succeed without concentrating all his confidence and dedication towards his goals. Will-power, belief and self-confidence will reap the results, nothing else.

Aristotle said that one can reach any destination with expectations in his mind and commitment in his heart. But the one who tries to achieve multiple goals simultaneously can never move forward. If we want we can definitely move ahead in life, but we have to be committed, consistent and repeat our efforts again and again so that it becomes a habit – and helps to grow our potential.

One can sharpen one's mind by using it effectively. And the mind can remain stable by a strong decision. It gains potential by belief. If these qualities are lacking, all other efforts will prove futile. So identify your power and believe that you can succeed, you will work for it and achieve success.

One can do the most difficult task only when one's mind is full of creativity. An empty mind can do nothing. On the other hand, passion and excitement can reap great results. Don't worry if you are poor; throw away these thoughts. Get up and believe in yourself. Keep your eye on your aim, gain confidence, and put in all your heart and effort. Then you will definitely succeed in your mission.

Faith and duty

Count Leo Tolstoy of Russia was not only a gifted writer, but a great visionary and thinker as well. He said, 'Neither hope nor superstition can be called faith.' We should work according to our capability. A farmer ploughs the field and a boatman sails the boat. They do not have the same reason behind their jobs. These people love to achieve their goal. They are hopeful, yet they do not work through inspiration but because it is their business. They have successfully linked their skills to their profession, without dreaming emptily. If a person understands his potential to work as a labor, carpenter, or any businessman, then he can work accordingly and be successful. One must work according to one's potential, interest and aptitude. This is a personal decision, and arises from self awareness.

Tolstoy said, 'Faith and duty are not separate issues but two names. The only difference they have is that duty is performed externally while faith is internal. The relation between humanity and eternity is called faith. And we walk on its path after being introduced to it. So, true faith can never be dumb, or go against knowledge.'

When we do something, we expect positive results. We hear about students failing in board exams committing suicide. Why do we forget that it is the outcome of our lack of effort?

Why don't we analyze our work procedure and find our shortcomings? We hide our mistakes and seek sympathy – but can't get it. Naturally it leads us to suicide. It is good to trust God and pray to succeed, but we should not forget to make the effort as well. We have to write the correct answer, God won't do that for us in the exam hall. How can we blame the Almighty? True faith means making the best of our potential and opportunities. Even God doesn't help lazy people, and the result has to be failure. As they say, 'God helps only those who help themselves.'

A saying goes such: 'Do your duty, don't worry about the results.' It does not mean that you should stop thinking about the result, but that one should not chase the result greedily. If work is incomplete, results cannot happen. So, one has to be patient with failure. No one becomes successful without facing failure at first – so one must be ready for it. We have to face many challenges in life, and we will either fail or succeed. But we must keep trying until we succeed. It is the rule of nature that one has to accept his defeat and fight back. The faith towards God teaches us to have a strong commitment and ward off anxiety. Anxiety is our enemy which throws our belief off balance. There is a saying, 'There is no other sin like disappointment. So, you should finish off this sinful act and become hopeful.'

Science and spirituality are inter-related to each other

Whereas spirituality is gaining success, science is also growing fast. We have proved all the matters of universe like planets, life, nature, etc., with scientific principles. If we research our holy books, we will find that science and spirituality were never different. These are two faces of the same coin. In fact, science is wide enough to include our religions and truths. But gradually, superstition separated from science. Today, it is spreading disease in our society. It is important to understand this. Dr. A P J Abdul Kalam wrote... 'This country cannot be empowered only by financial stability. Its foundation rests on its values and principles. And it needs scientific direction. Combining the two is the best way one can emerge as a superpower. Every kind of knowledge can be imparted through scientific methods, and can enable our faith, trust, confidence and belief in God to advance and grow'.

An inspirational magazine wrote, 'We can direct human life with the help of education. Combination of education and science can enrich and fuel one's life. If education is physical, then science is spiritual. We have to know both. It can open the doors of progress and help us compete with other nations. Science should not dominate us, so it is important to know religion too. One should not have blind faith in spirituality, so science should be taught with it. One can be successful in this 21st century by knowing the evidences of science and adopting the knowledge of spirituality.'

Our country has always been a mine of scientific thought. This is the reason we have produced great scientists and invented marvelous products. Newton hoped to know about the universe. He found ways to reach different parts of universe to know their secrets. He researched on the topics written in the holy books. Saints never separated science from spirituality. Science is an important part of our life. If science is supportive in physical inventions, then spirituality plays the same role in mental pleasures. Spiritual power is a kind of waterfall that has no source but it can't be hidden. James Allen conceived this as the best form of spirituality.

He said, 'Living a life of love and affection is the true meaning of life.'

Spirituality is defined in a manner that it is too far removed from our daily work, but has all the sources of work. It is the storehouse of all knowledge and inspiration. Science and spirituality seem to be different, but actually, are same. We have to learn spirituality in order to know science. There is no clash between them. Accept to combine them and you will find the solution.

❑

3

HOPE & CONFIDENCE

- *Be optimistic*
- *Doors to success*
- *Winning fuss*
- *Discard your anxiety*
- *Hope and confidence*
- *Know your inner potential*
- *Self-confidence is the basis of all potential*
- *Believe in yourself*
- *Hope and enthusiasm*
- *Be a firm believer while studying*

Be optimistic

Allen, a famous thinker, said, 'One who is optimistic can be successful. When there is no hope, there can be no success.' Hope has a unique power to bring on confidence, creativity and the potential to succeed in a person. Those who are optimists have enormous creative powers. They are highly capable and have immense happiness inside. But the pessimist has no energy or potential. He keeps on worrying about success and failure, and ends up doing nothing.

Until we have the confidence to achieve our goals, we cannot succeed in any exam. But confidence and hope can help us succeed powerfully. Charles said, 'I have observed that successful people are always happy and hopeful. They initiate all tasks with happiness and positive enthusiasm, which brings a glow to their face, and they take advantage of it to succeed. They bear and fight all problems strongly and remain calm.'

Manavasyon sarwa saphalyam jivanasya cha,
Charitartha tatha srishterashavade pratitishthim.

Man's success and progress lies in his attitude and optimism. Hope has the power to bring confidence and inspires us to move ahead in life. Many great men have won due to hope. They became an inspiration for others. Henry Ford, Edison, etc., never lost hope and continued to work even when they failed many times, and ultimately conquered success.

Hope and worry are two faces of life. A hopeful person does not lack courage and ability. These people are governed by their confidence which inspires them to make continuous efforts and succeed in life. Negative thinkers are always doubtful about results and become cowards. They lose their ability to think and cannot identify the path of success.

We know that God helps those who help themselves. One writer states, 'When you always tend to succeed in life, then it becomes natural for you to believe in your inner self. It keeps you confident and helps you zoom into new ways and paths of success everytime. Gradually, you begin believing that God is there to show you the right path. He instills confidence in your mind and you use it to move on the right path. You never hesitate to move ahead.' But those who have no confidence are doubtful about every task. They cannot take any firm decision and remain indecisive. They do not believe they can succeed in life and thus they cannot begin any task. They should start hoping or at least think about how one could succeed, and become happy? In reality, we can escape from disappointment through our confidence. All we need is to make an effort to make our life beautiful. When you are attracted by any material thing, you tend to get it by any means, and you have to believe that you will achieve it. Someone has rightly said, 'It is not only important to dream about something, but one should have intense desire to achieve it as well.' It means that if you think and believe with a strong desire, then you can definitely achieve your goals.

Belief is really important. It is the secret to succeed in life, to reach your destination. Whosoever has succeeded in this world had gathered and channelized all his mental and physical energy to use it to gain success. They faced many obstacles but fought courageously and never doubted their potential and never gave up. Their hope enabled them to win and showed them the doors to success.

Doors to success

Vidur, the wise man in Mahabharata, explained the difference between an intelligent person and a fool as, 'Intelligent is one who chooses the best goal and never focuses on critics. Anger, ego and humiliation cannot harm him. What he wants, he creates himself. Climatic variations, financial instability or physical barriers cannot stop him. He works according to his potential and never wastes time. It is the mark of an intelligent mind which decides very carefully, and never cries for what he has not achieved. He is not scared of problems and knows how to benefit from the lessons of hard times. He is not overly pleased by respect, and not overly saddened by insult. He knows how to carry himself, and be courteous and responsible in society. He works meticulously and accepts the truth.'

About fools, Vidur said, 'The one who dreams big in spite of being incapable, wants results without efforts, is a fool. The one who always interferes with others' jobs and forgets his own, is a fool. He is for ever postponing work, and feels too lazy to complete it on time. He criticizes others, and overlooks his own shortcomings. He is lazy, but always busy – with the wrong things.'

Some principles in life can make us successful or unsuccessful. This is a truth and those who refuse to believe it fail in life. Today's world is fiercely competitive. People are more worried of others' success than their own failures. They want more, but do less. It increases their dissatisfaction. But those who are satisfied move ahead with hard work. They achieve all their goals in life. We should not think wrongly about others and be supportive to all. We have to change our thoughts and attitude. Everyone gets results according to his capability. Some get it sooner, others later. So, one should work with dedicated efforts. Dissatisfied people should look at themselves, assess their potential realistically and build their life accordingly. This way, they will be able to succeed in life.

Orison Swett Marden said, 'You can be satisfied in your life, no matter what you do, and gain peace through it. You need to create interest in your work and contribute to it. The same task has the power to either create dissatisfaction in one's mind or bring peace. All he needs to do change is his attitude towards a more positive one. You can have peace in all walks of life. There will be problems and obstacles and you will feel lost, but you have to conquer them and move ahead towards your goals. When you take one positive step during your problems, you will find peace in it. It cannot be explained, but can be experienced. No route of life is devoid of problems, and it is not possible to reach your target without difficulties.'

Every one has to face difficulties in life. This is the rule of nature. Problems surround us to examine our potential. We have to think that we have to win. Do not let negativity dominate your mind. If you think your job is tough, then fight back with all your potential and beat it. Difficulties are tough when you are weak inside. A weak mind is a dangerous place. We have to fight every obstacle. Khalil Gibran said, 'Problems arise not from incompletion of a task. It is a sign of incompleteness and inadequacy. So, it must be conquered. The solutions can be found out and understood well. It is true that one must walk the road of failure, in order to succeed. One has to see poverty to be rich. Thus, we should not forget that problems are the doors to our success. One can achieve it only through efforts.'

Winning fuss

Nagarjuna, the famous Ayurvedic scholar, had to select a disciple. His students visited him one Thursday to show him their talent. Nagarjuna wanted a true candidate, so he selected two candidates for the final competition. He said, 'I will test you and make one of you my disciple.'

The next day, he handed over some material to them and asked for a solution. He gave them two days to finish the task. They appeared after two days but only one was carrying the solution. Nagarjuna asked him, 'Did you not face any problem while solving it?' The candidate replied, 'I faced problems. My mother was ill and I could not bring the medicine for her. My father had stomach-ache and my younger brother was injured. He was crying in pain, but I could not help them, because I had to make this.'

Nagarjuna smiled, then turned to the second candidate, who had brought no solution. He said, 'I am sorry for not being able to complete the task.' Nagarjuna asked the reason for it. He replied, 'I did not have any problem, but did my duty. I found a poor old man on the way and took him to my house. I spent my whole time looking after him… and I had no time left to make the solution.'

Nagarjuna asked the first candidate to go back home, and selected the second one. The first candidate said, 'How can you select the one who doesn't have a solution, and reject me, who has a solution?' Nagarjuna replied, 'The solution is supposed to be a life saver. Your priority was to save a life. But you put your parent's and brother's life in danger, while this boy helped save the old man's life. Therefore, I have selected the person who truly fulfilled his duty.'

There is no person who has not faced problems or will have no problems ahead in the future. Every one has to face problems in life. We feel disappointed with problems and we forget that one who fights, wins. It is said, 'The easiest way to escape from problems is to keep away from feelings of negativity and fear. Never worry about the load you have to carry. Think whether your task is really difficult. Imagine your problem as a test to prove your capability. What is pain? Confucius said, 'Hey fool, man's doubt is pain, lack of knowledge is load.' Throw away your doubts and selfishness, and behave like a carefree person. Your problems will be eliminated. Lack of knowledge brings doubts, and you feel sad. So, fight your problems and you will succeed.'

People generally become sad in difficult times and say, 'I am very unhappy, what should I do?' or 'I am in an unusual problem'. We know that no one is going to help us, yet we talk about it. Hence, it is better to find a solution to your problem than crying about it. You will have to find the solution yourself and gain your confidence back. Be focused and you will find the solution.

Discard your anxiety

We become tense when we face challenges. This is natural, and it could be either dangerous or helpful. If you are fearful of your challenges and doubt your talent, then it can harm you. On the other hand, if you make consistent efforts to face your challenge head on and tackle your problems, it can help you succeed.

In the face of a challenge, we have to be patient and persistent in order to find the solution. If we doubt or fear our capabilities, then the solution will elude us. Our stability is endangered by the uneasiness of our mind. Our thoughts start wandering and we become indecisive. Why does this happen? A thinker wrote, 'A big part of the human community surrenders to anxiety. As a result, we doubt our plans. We focus too much on the obstacles, and are unable to sleep at night, and are disturbed during the day. Fear scares us and pushes us towards failure. On the other hand, if a person remains calm and focused and happy, he can work on his plan and tackle every problem and move towards his goal.

Some people get influenced by other people's words, and fear needlessly. They have doubts before taking an exam, or appearing for an interview – this weakens their confidence. The more you worry, the bigger the problem becomes. We fail and do not understand the root cause of it. It is said that 'Worrying is a fool's game. The more we worry, the weaker we become. These people invite problems at every step.'

Actually, one needs to concentrate. If your mind is full of doubts and fears, then it cannot accomplish any task. One needs to be fearless in order to work. Creativity arises from focus. If we fear or doubt ourselves, then we are igniting the fuel of failure. We weaken our potential and this takes us away from our path. A thinker said, 'When the mind is doubtful, it cannot do a job effectively.' So, we should keep away our fear so that we may fight the challenges with a steady mind. Doubt multiplies fear and weakens us. It blocks the flow of creative thoughts in our minds, and reduces our capacity to work effectively. Whenever you are surrounded by fear, always let it flow out of your system and invite new and positive ones in their place, instead. Emotional feelings have immense power which can bring great results. An old lady said 'I have made it a habit to hope for good. When I wake up, I believe my day to be best day of my life. I go for a new journey everyday.' So, worrying about the unknown and harassing our own minds is useless. We entrap ourselves more and more into it, and become weaker than before. Henry Ward Beecher, a social reformer, said, 'One does not die from work, but from worrying about it.' One remains healthy by work, and this is the secret of success.

Hope and confidence

One of the most renowned Hindi poets, Maithilisharan Gupta said, '*Nar ho, na nirash karo man ko* (You are a man, do not depress yourself).' This inspires us to be optimistic. Great men have experienced that the impossible becomes possible only when a person moves ahead with passion and persistence. Hope provides energy to be successful on the journey.

Bhartrihari writes, 'Hope is like a river where the water of wishes flow. Its waves are desires and demands act like crocodiles. Worry is its bank, reasons are its birds and those who move along its trees of patience, find everlasting peace in life.'

Hope provides us the energy to move ahead in life. There is no problem in life that cannot be solved. Every problem has a solution. All one needs is commitment and dedication.

This thought arises only when one thinks about it. He has to believe that he can win and achieve his goals. The one who is depressed loses his track even before starting out. Be patient and excited - Never give in to depression. If you fall prey to hopelessness, you will not be able to accomplish anything great in life.

Mahatma Gandhi said, 'Hope is eternal, its application never fails.' A hopeful person always thinks positively, and remains calm and happy in every situation - and therefore succeeds in life. An optimist retains his confidence in every situation and gains success in every task.

Social thinker John Ruskin said, 'If the heart goes down, life goes down'. There is nothing except loss of enthusiasm which can create trouble for a human being. The image of hope is blurred when it is surrounded by doubts. The expectations begin to die and one takes recourse to the path of failure. Thus, a positive thought is the parameter and determining factor of one's success. It is power in the true sense, which can defeat any one in this world. An optimist can never be defeated and nothing can damage him. So, stay away from depression and succeed with hope.

Orison Swett Marden said, 'Hope and confidence are the two essential qualities that bring energy to win, and multiply it every time.' Shivaji was famous for his towering presence in the battle field, and his soldiers gained confidence through it. His majestic leadership motivated and energized them. Shivaji won battles because he had never known, or tasted, defeat...

Someone has very rightly said, 'The little rays of hope in the darkness have immense importance in life than we can realize.' When we are surrounded by problems, we need hope to win, to succeed, to come out of a difficult situation. If there is confidence, the ray of hope will definitely appear, get brighter gradually, and lead us to the solution.

There was a poor villager whose father had died. The child, inspired by his mother, started selling soaps. Gradually, one day, he became the owner of a soap factory. So instead of being discouraged by his father's death, he chose to take his mother's route of inspiration and hard work. Thus, optimism is a thought, and an inner light, that keeps us happy, removes our fears, and relieves us of pain.

Know your inner potential

A thinker has said, 'The moment a person decides to complete a task, the job is as good as done. Weak people used to boast of like Shekh Chilli but a committed person shows it in his results.'

We have enough energy inside us to perform miracles, but we need to identify it first. A thinker writes, 'A huge tree has its power in a small seed. This seed becomes gigantic with time and manure. Similarly, humans have enormous power inside them. They too can identify it and become great like others, all they need is to use it carefully. If he uses his potential on the right path, it can roll out the world at his feet and everyone would be amazed to see that.'

We should believe in our potential and our confidence makes our potential grow. It teaches us to live happily. Remember, our belief connects our potential to God and opens the doors to success. Belief neither thinks nor guesses. It only knows to believe and engenders confidence in us. All the energies inside our body converge and explode like dynamite, fuelling us towards success. Lack of confidence is our greatest enemy.

Orison Swett Marden has written, 'All the problems, failures, etc., in life are due to lack of belief. Tell yourself 'I am a child of God. God does not accept a weak mind. He has made me to win, not to lose. He never makes anyone fail.'

So, one can be inspired by linking oneself to God; this generates confidence within us. Generate positive thoughts in your mind. Become your own true friend and you can become great. A French general told his soldiers, 'We have no right to be called humans until we gain victory over every problem and earn the capability to succeed. One cannot succeed without self-confidence. This cycle of the universe is very well governed. It teaches us the secrets of success. One has to sow the seed to reap the fruits. Your talent and potential are all a waste if you lack confidence. You cannot reap the benefit of any of these powerful qualities unless you have confidence.'

Until we apply all our potential to a job and concentrate on it, we do not accomplish any task. The more difficult a task, the more passion and efforts it requires. God helps those who help themselves. So, remember the secret of success is confidence.

Self-confidence is the basis of all potential

Listen to this fairy tale. There was once a saint named Shaumya. A student named Aruni appeared in his ashram. The Guru wanted to test him on the very first day. It was raining heavily and the guru asked him 'Son, go and check the dam; and if there is any crack in it, plug the hole and tie it properly.'

The boy went to the field and analyzed the dam closely, and found a leakage. He kept applying mud on it and tried to stop the leakage. But suddenly, the water broke the mud wall, and came gushing out. Aruni decided to lie down in the path of the gushing water, creating a human instead.

Back at the ashram, it was getting dark and Aruni had not returned yet. Shaumya started to get worried, and so he went to the field with his students and searched for Aruni. He found him unconscious at the mud wall. They took him back to the ashram and helped him recover. This confidence and dedication impressed his guru very much. Aruni came to be respected the most among all the students.

This story is an example of belief and dedication. Work is worship. Whatever we have to do, whether it is studying, job, business, etc., we should be dedicated to it. This dedication brings confidence in us and inspires us to succeed; it never lets us detour from the right path. People who follow this golden rule never fail in life. This dedication makes our confidence grow and enables us to gain an edge over others. Swami Rama Tirtha said, 'There is no need to stand outside the earth to destroy it, but you need confidence, self-confidence. One can create miracles with its power and most of our troubles disappear by its force. Those who apply it in life, never fail.

Our confidence allows us to fight the most difficult of obstacles. A thinker has written, 'The basis of our energy is confidence. In its shortage, one can become 'unconscious' without even realizing it. As it grows, other powers also grow with it together, they drive us powerfully to explore life along its many directions, and succeed. All impossible tasks become possible and we become super humans.' One should remember that nothing is impossible with self-confidence. Someone said, 'A man needs to keep working on his thoughts and refine them regularly. He should improve by keeping selfishness away, and by being 'content'. So, one should have dedication, belief and passion in him. No one can then stop him from being successful. The whole world becomes his.

Believe in yourself

You must have read the stories of *Panchtantra* by Pandit Vishnu Sharma. He used to teach the sons of kings and nobles. He wrote these stories to teach them discipline, intelligence, etc. One day, he was playing with his students when his friends arrived. They were surprised and asked him, 'Vishnu, why are you playing with kids? You are wasting your precious time.' Vishnu Sharma murmured something into his student's ear and the kid brought a bow from inside. Vishnu handed it to his friend and said, 'This is the issue. Can you solve it?' His friend could not understand him. Vishnu replied, 'Our mind is like a bow. If it is tied tightly both ways, it will break. But if it is relaxed for a while, then it will be ok. If our heart is stressed, it will break, and we will fall ill. All work and no play does not ensure success; in fact, it endangers it.'

The one who trusts his potential, soul and talent succeeds in life. We should remember that ambition becomes more powerful with proper self-examination. Your efforts are just like your thoughts... and the way you think affects your life every moment, in every way. A thinker has said, 'If your mind is weak, unstable and feeble, you cannot accomplish any task. Petty thoughts lead to petty results. We need to identify our potential and work according to it. Great personalities of the world have sacrificed their lives to achieve their goals.'

You might have read the idiom, 'You reap what you sow' – it applies everywhere. A person becomes like his thoughts. So, think according to your ideals. Believe in yourself that you will succeed and you will actually succeed. You have to keep on trying and believing in yourself.

An old man was planting trees in a garden when the king approached him. He saw his dedication and asked 'What are you doing?' The man replied, 'I am planting mango trees.' The king asked, 'Do you know you won't be able to reap the fruits because you are too old?' The old man said, 'I know I won't be alive, but it is for the next generation. I am a giver, not a taker.' The king was impressed and rewarded him with gold coins. The man said, 'See, I have reaped the fruits right now!'

You should do your work sincerely and you will accomplish your goal. Whatever you do, you will face circumstances that are in favour or against you, but when you focus your energies, the sky is the limit!

Banish the thought that only the rich, or those with resources, succeed. Don't get into the trap of thinking about talent, connections and fate – all that you need to succeed is already in you. You have to identify your true potential and nurture it, and you will definitely succeed.

Hope and enthusiasm

Lady Merry was a hard working lady in America. She was widowed at the age of 18 and was illiterate. But she wanted to achieve something in life so she learned painting. She started making natural paintings. She used to earn little from her paintings but she never complained and continued to work with enthusiasm. Gradually, she started earning more and more, and attained great levels of success. She established a Trust to help women and continued her painting right till her last days. Today, she is an example of hope and enthusiasm for everyone.

Orison Swett Marden said, 'Hope and self-confidence can give rise to enormous energy which multiplies your potential.' The one who works with hope and enthusiasm succeeds in life. Those who think that they will not succeed, never start anything in life. They are forever surrounded by anxiety and have no enthusiasm. Their dynamism breaks down and, not surprising, they fail. So, remember the shloka:

Utsaho balvanarya nastayutshatparam balam,
Sotsahasya hi lokeshu na kinchidapi durlabham.

It means that enthusiasm is the strongest force in the planet, and there is nothing stronger than it. Nothing is too difficult for an enthusiastic person.

Hope and enthusiasm can turn defeat into victory, failure into success and negativity into positivity. We need to have such an attitude. It provides the confidence to overcome any difficulty. The one who possesses this energy cannot be defeated. The one who is sailing in the boat of negativity can never reach his destination. John Ruskin said, 'I know nothing except hope and enthusiasm, which can be essential for success.' When there is no enthusiasm there are no results.

Hope gives inspiration to move ahead in life. Hope is life and life is hope. But if they are not linked together, they can be of no use. Inspiration is useful when applied. These are all interconnected; If one link breaks, the other also gets weakened. Munshi Premchand has rightly said, 'Hope is the creator of excitement. It has power, life and passion inside it. It governs our lives.' All we need to do is work efficiently, and success will be ours.

There was a kid, Kilonthis. He was studying in Geno's school. He was a poor guy and hardly had any clothes to wear. He worked and also started studying in school. He paid the fee everyday and studied. One day, his rich friends came to know the reality, and got jealous. They started calling him poor and a thief. They complained against him in school and talked ill of him to their own families. Their parents called the police and the boy was arrested. He was taken to court. He called two witnesses to help him prove his innocence. The first person was a gardener. He said that the boy worked in his garden and earned a little amount from him. The other witness was an old lady who replied, 'This boy visits my house every week and does some household work, and I pay him.' His innocence was proved and he was acquitted. The judge was impressed and offered to pay his fees. But the boy refused by saying, 'I am honest and hard working. I will earn and pay my own fees.' Everyone felt ashamed about themselves on hearing this.

Manavsyonnati sarva safalyam jivanasya cha,
Charitarthya tatha srishteshavade pratishthitam.

It means that the seeds to life's success lies in one's character.

Be a firm believer while studying

Every exam, big or small, is a challenge where we have to produce our best. One must possess the inner confidence and the patience to succeed, even though it may not be evident outside to others. There is hardly any person who has not been tested by God. We have many examples and anecdotes in our holy books and scriptures telling us how saints and devas of old had to undergo severe tests and challenges in their lives. There is competition in everyone's life. Sage Vishwamitra tested Raja Harishchandra and in the end, Raja Harishchandra won over Sage Vishwamitra and all the Gods, and was ensured a place in heaven. We know that we have to go through fire to glitter like gold.

Rishi Mudgal was a famous saint. He was very poor. His family could barely afford one square in a day, sometimes even less. One day, as they were preparing for their meal, a guest arrived unexpectedly. They were worried: What can we offer to our guest? The guest asked, 'Where is Mudgal? I want to share a meal with him.' Mudgal welcomed him and said, 'I was waiting for you. Please have a seat.' As Mudgal served, the guest kept eating, and finished all the food. It was 15 days ago that he and his family had had a meal last. Even on this day, his family had to make do with water, but on this day, they broke down and fell ill.

A few days later, Mudgal visited saint Durvasa's ashram, and invited him over again. Durvasa replied, 'I had disguised myself as your guest to test you. You have succeeded in the exam.'

We should not be scared of tests and should keep our cool. Those who do not fear problems say, 'God is testing us'. Vedvyas said:

Datushavaiv pariksha vai durbhikshe cha jayte nirbhi,
Shurasyaiv tu sangrame mitrasya cha tathapadi.
Ashaktao cha tatha strina vipatto sukulasya cha,
Snehasya cha parokshen satasya sankate gate.

God's test in prayer, brave's in war, friend is tested in emergency, lady in poverty, a good family in hardship, love in arrogance and truth is tested in trouble.

We have to be committed to our task. We should fine-tune and focus all our inner potential and produce our best. Those who are scared of tests cannot triumph in life. A test should be like a routine task. Those who prepare well for it are not scared by it. But those who are depressed never prepare well, and fail. So, fight with confidence and gain enthusiasm to emerge as the best. You will surely succeed. This confidence should remain in you during your trying times.

❑

④

SELF-ACKNOWLEDGEMENT

- *Self-acknowledgement is the best knowledge*
- *Never trust fate*
- *Analyze yourself*
- *Throw away your negativity*
- *Be quiet at times*
- *Our character is our success*
- *Believe yourself, know yourself*
- *Know your inner potiential*

Self-acknowledgement is the best knowledge

The famous Greek philosopher Socrates stated, 'Know your self.' He wrote it on the front door of a temple. He did it so that every visitor begins to understand and accept his own self. It was his experience that our achievements and art of living depends on our self acknowledgement. Thus, every one should know about himself before commencing any task. It actually indicates that we can achieve our targets by knowing our potential. One should not become over confident and take wrong steps in any walk of life; otherwise, one faces heavy defeat, and ends up blaming others for their failure. The reason is that we do not 'know' or trust ourselves and expect more out of our efforts. But the truth is that we are really not aware of ourselves and our true potential. You can be overpowering and have the qualities of a successful person if you start acknowledging yourself. Some people are quick to learn this, while others take a long time. But you should have the desire to know yourself.

It is said in the Bible that we resemble God. It means that we should be qualitative, talented, a forgiver and eternal. We have the potential to be like Him. But the root of our trouble is that we hardly use our potential to the fullest. Scientists say that the human uses only 20% of his brain, maybe even less. Just think – if you are an average person and using 20%, then what in life could you achieve if you use 100% of your brain power. You already have all the potential - you simply need to open the locks of that potential. A person should be like a waterfall - continuously flowing and in motion. You are, then, capable of fighting any challenge and moving forward.

When Henry Ford succeeded in inventing the Model-T, America's most popular economical car, he could have hung up his boots. But he did not stop there. He kept on researching to make better cars to make them accessible to everyone. The Wright Brothers gave us the gift of flight by inventing the first aeroplane, but they had to overcome various obstacles and repetitive failures before attaining success. They controlled their minds and gained the energy to succeed. Winning was natural for them, because when one realizes and uses his potential to the fullest, no power on Earth can stop him from succeeding. We should never think that we are weak. Rather, you must say to yourself that you are capable, and you will experience that you have gained self-confidence, and that it is driving you towards success.

Vedvyas wrote in the *Mahabbharata* - 'Self knowledge is the best knowledge.' Socrates recognized this talent and wrote on walls of a temple 'The one who does not know himself does not know God'. The Buddhist Dhammpad says, 'The one who knows himself won't go and teach others.' Swami Rama Tirtha explains it 'Self acknowledgement is the first and foremost duty of a human being.' We should know ourselves to succeed in life. Gautam Buddha said, 'One who can control himself cannot be defeated by anyone.'

Never trust fate

People who fail in exams, are rejected in interviews or fail in business, say one word - 'Bad-luck'. There is a huge hue and cry about fate, astrology, and similar things. People take it for granted and say, 'Be calm and your days will be back; you will soon be happy, your time is yet to come.' And some people also believe, 'When one is lucky, he will have success at his doorstep.' Malookdas said 'Cobra never bites, birds never chirp; It is God who controls us all.' We stop finding solutions by blaming our fate and live a life of negativity. If we are lucky enough we will get it - this attitude is endless and pointless, and should be rejected. It drags you towards failure and teaches you to be lazy. Those who use their confidence and potential to win fight bravely and succeed in their mission. Society runs on the drive and courage of such winning personalities.

Dependency on fate drags us to failure. It makes us static and lazy. The Gita inspires us by teaching us to not think about results, and to simply focus on our duty ('karma'). Every society, every community changes with time and we have to change with it. We can create our future on the foundation of the past and build our present to have a secure future ahead. The past can never be the future. Our ancestors have talked about fate and duty, and it is still followed by us. However, the way our values are changing sharply, we need to grow and evolve with it, else we will lag behind. Science has advanced incredibly in recent times, and constantly reminds us to stay away from fate, luck and charm, and advices us to work hard. Swami Ram Tirth said, 'Man is the creator of his destiny.' He inspires us to refrain from being dependent on luck. Valmiki said that luck is that which cannot be visualized and decided by human beings. Only cowards believe in luck.

Those who 'gives themselves up' to fate should be ready to fail – God also tells us the same. He wants to say that let the secret of failure be a secret. Do not waste your time and energy trying to 'discover' it. Complete your tasks properly and never think about the results. One person reached God and saw God writing people's fate. The man asked God to tell him their fate, so that he could help them by telling them their own fates. But God refused by saying, 'It would be dramatically worthless to tell them their fate.' On being asked the reason, God replied, 'Those who know that their fate is not in their favour will not work hard, because they will think that they would not be successful, so what's the use of working anyway? People who are not so lazy will become lazy too, because of the same reasons. And thus everyone in this world would become lazy and never make any effort to do anything. In truth, one never reaps results without hard work, and this is one central rule of life that I cannot break. Hence, let things be as they are. Don't ask me anymore. Those who assure by predicting your fate and future don't actually know it – they deceive and befool you all.'

Someone has correctly said, 'Luck sleeps when you are not working, and works for you when you begin your task.' In reality, there is no luck that falls from the sky onto your lap. An astrologer cannot bring you luck. Luck is the result of your efforts and you will receive it accordingly. If you do not work hard, there is no power that can reap the results for you. The tree grows only when the seed is planted and nurtured properly with sunlight, water and manure. The truth is that characterisation and imagination builds your fate. According to Roman poet Virgil, 'Luck favours only brave men.' Vivekananda said, 'Bury your past and your future will be in front of you. Remember to work hard and make your luck work for you.'

Analyze yourself

One day, a gold coin was kept with waste papers in the dust-bin. The proud coin saw them and said in anger and contempt, "Oh you dirty papers, I am being irritated by you! Go away from here; I am a gold coin.' The papers were quiet and did not argue. After some days, the papers were taken out and supplied to a paper mill where they were transformed into currency notes. Each paper now amounted to around 10 gold coins. When the money was being counted, the gold coin was present there, and felt ashamed. The papers said, 'Your ego never does you any good. Never call anyone unimportant. Anyone can become great with time. Ego is not useful for anyone.'

Thus, you can bid goodbye to your bad habits by analyzing yourself and separately 'highlighting' those qualities that can help you reach great heights. Nobody knows us better than ourselves. But we should consult others to know what they feel about us so that we may abandon our bad habits. Ego is a bad habit that affects us badly. A person who is full of ego has a disease that makes him feel well, but makes others sick. We keep on repeating 'I did it, I am the doer, executor and so on.' The British priest Colton said, 'Ego is like a magnet which attracts from one side but repels from the other side. People try to belittle others with their potential and in this practice they keep them away from themselves. They keep on making mistakes while considering their mistakes as their achievements.' It is a sign of selfishness, conceit and short-sightedness that clouds one's reasoning and drowns one in failure. Everyone thinks better about himself and challenges others. Instead of supporting others, we try to pull them down.

We should understand the meaning of 'the self'. It is always a respectable and honest identity of a person. But it does not mean that one should adopt ego in his behavior. A person should be polite and natural. Our culture teaches us to be polite and humble to all. Therefore, our 'self' is a beautiful term and not a part of ego. One should leave behind his ego and not his 'self'. Ego is like a balloon which can burst anytime without prior warning. Hence, we need to be aware of it and all those who possess it. Ego is an illusion that shatters the learning power of your brain and takes you to the wrong path, considering it right. The one who does not understand this concept can never grow in life. Our essence is our culture, traditions, values and beliefs which are respected by others, but ego does not allow our essence to sparkle and shine. Only ego can take you towards failure, and destroy you, your personality and your future.

British writer John Ruskin writes, 'An egotist is deep into the channels of blunders'. Lord Vishnu appointed Jai and Vijay as his gatekeepers, and they were super egotists. They knew nobody could enter without their permission, so they stopped everyone from meeting the Lord. One day, they stopped goddess Lakshmi and were very pleased with themselves. She cursed them to become demons, and they were later reborn as Ravan-Kumbhkaran, Hirnayakashyap and Shishupal-Duryodhan. Therefore, when ego comes in the way it destroys everyone.

Throw away your negativity

Once a man approached a shoemaker to repair his shoe. The shoemaker refused to stitch the shoe because it was time to close the shop. The man said, 'If you don't stitch my shoe, then I will be left with only one shoe, so please repair it.' But the shoemaker did not agree and said, 'You can have my shoe.' The man replied, 'I do not wear other's shoes and the shoemaker asked, 'If you can exchange your thoughts, then why not the shoes?' The other person was left speechless. It is true that we exchange knowledge with others whether it is positive or negative. If we absorb positive thoughts, we reap good results and succeed in life, while negative thoughts can only lead to bad results. We also make our children pessimists by saying, 'Nothing will happen, this is useless.'

We have to be alert that our thoughts and actions are affecting others, thus these should be positive. We will have to grow our confidence and keep away from negative thinkers. Remember, negative thoughts never let us move ahead. It is better to absorb good thoughts and apply them in life. Those who want to be the best, work for the best – and we all want the best in life. Therefore, don't be negative.

Some people try to adopt the policy of 'if', but do not make the necessary efforts. These people say, 'If I had done this, if I had done that' and then regret. They are never active. On the other hand, positive thinkers just work hard and achieve their goals. They are confident and have well-defined and clear goals. They are never disappointed by challenges and fight courageously.

Swami Sukhbodhananda says, 'We should learn to analyze ourselves and never put negative thoughts in our mind. Some thoughts are our enemies and we have to analyze ourselves to keep away from such thoughts. If we don't stop this flow, then it will ruin our life. So, choose the best for yourself.'

It is true that the direction of life depends on our thoughts. If we choose the wrong direction, then we will be pessimistic in life and have negative outcomes. On the contrary, if we choose the better, positive side, then success will be ours. You will experience that positive thoughts have positive energy and everything becomes possible with it. Life becomes satisfactory and miraculous. Everything happens for the good, but we make it poor by our thoughts. Unfortunately, we do not identify the hidden values of life because it has a layer of speculative clouds. If you understand the underlying values and power of life, then it can be a boon for you. Swami Sukhbodhananda says, 'Watch a honey bee; it collects the honey from each flower and brings it to its place. But the common bee sits on dirt and brings dust and disease with it. We are surrounded by diseases; hence positive thoughts should be absorbed by you (like the honey bee) and negative ones thrown away (like the ordinary bee). This will definitely steer your life in the right direction.'

Be quiet at times

There were two friends who went out in search of a mentor. They reached a forest and found a saint in a hut. They greeted him and asked him for help. The saint was quiet and just watched them patiently. But the boys doubted the saint's abilities as he was not answering them. One thought, 'Either he is an egotist, or he does not have knowledge. He might be having tremendous potential, but does not think that we deserve his advice.' They left. Later on in life, one of the two friends became an egotist while the other became polite and humble. The humble person approached the saint after a few years and said, 'You explained us every thing on that day by being quiet. I have understood that we lacked the politeness and etiquette in our lives, hence I worked upon it. I have understood the value of silence and have observed changes in my life.'

In reality, it is very important to consider carefully the words that we speak and to whom we are speaking. Most people are so talkative that they do not know when to stop speaking once they start, and as a result end up speaking badly about others, which harms them later on.

A thinker said, 'Many people are in the habit of talking and keep their tongues in motion. They can not resist speaking even when it is not required. They are not aware of the power associated with each word they speak. We have to remember that crossing the limits can be the cause of arguments. But the one who speaks well becomes the centre of attraction in society.' It is said 'Speak little, speak well.' When one utters a sound, he instils life into his speech. But a harsh tone of speech will always bring about rage and resentment, raise your blood pressure, and increase the chances of disease and bitter feelings. So, it is better to speak less than to speak evil.

Silence can be helpful to us when we do not want to reply or are not sure of our answer. Our silence does not leave a negative impact on others. The other benefit is that we get time to think when we observe silence and speak with better knowledge. Kabir says:

'Vad vivad vish ghana, bole bahut upadh,

Maun gahe sabki sahe, sumire naam agadh.

Arguments only create trouble in life and one can never win an argument. Thinkers have advised us to express our feelings in little, well thought out words as it will not leave a bad impression on others. One thinker says, 'A talkative person leaves an insignificant and fleeting impression on others and hence he should think before speaking.' Gandhiji spent most of his time in silence. He would speak only when it was required. He said, 'I feel peaceful when I am mute and refresh my mind with silence. It is Godly to practice silence in daily life.'

There was a saint – Bhashkali who approached his mentor's ashram. During a conversation, he asked, 'Sir, tell me the secret of the universe.' The mentor was quiet and Bhashkali kept repeating the question. At last he asked, 'Are you not satisfied with my question?' The mentor replied, 'I have replied you many times, but you did not understand. One cannot learn about the universe by hearing or saying; you have to understand it with silence.'

There is only one way for self-improvement and self-analysis in life, and it is silence. Self-improvement and self-analysis direct our life, and aid us in finding solutions to our problems. It also enhances our character and helps us tackle our difficulties.

Our character is our success

German philosopher Friedrich Wilhelm Nietzsche said, 'Bad character is always stained.' It means that our character is the foundation of our success. If there is no impact of our character on others, then it is worthless. It will not help anyone to succeed in society. Charles Schwab says, 'The character of a person is like the fragrance of a flower.' As the fragrance of a flower adds to its charm, the character of a person makes him meaningful and enriched. Leading Hindi writer Bhagwati

Charan Verma wrote, 'There are few personalities that attract others like a magnet.'

Once, Shivaji attacked Ballari with his small battalion and defeated them easily. Ballari's queen was also imprisoned and Shivaji ordered to present the queen to him. The queen said, 'I feel insulted when you respect me. You must treat me like a defeated enemy.' Shivaji was astonished with the queen's personality, and his respect and admiration for her grew. He approached the queen and greeted her by saying 'You deserve respect from all. My mother has expired recently and I can see her reflection in your personality. I'll always treat you like my mother.' The queen was also impressed by his words and started crying. She said, 'You are a true Maratha and will serve our nation with pride and distinction.'

Wealth and health were the only main constituents of one's personality in earlier times. A wealthy person was considered smart, even if he was ugly or lunatic. Gradually, people started getting attracted towards intelligence and the demand for education grew. People who were educated became the new status symbols of society. All we need to do is to enhance the growth of our character with education. Parents inculcate these habits in children. Character cannot be obtained or bought – it has to be built. Lilli Allen wrote, 'No one can defame you or build your character. You can be lunatic or wise, successful or unsuccessful. You can be anything and everything, or could be nothing; it is up to you. Don't worry about who you are – Just trust yourself and take a strong decision to grow in life.'

Your character is the true image of your personality. If you don't have a sound character and have a mind clouded with jealousy and negative thoughts, it will be reflected in your work and behaviour. It also affects you (and others) in other ways. In today's world, one may befriend a politician; but they often complain about them behind their backs. In general, people respect them even after knowing the reality and this puts them into more trouble. Lilli Allen writes 'The one who has sound character is honest and brave, and never gives in to adverse or ill-temptations. This type of person does not need a path, he creates one of his own. Admiration awaits this person and intelligence is eager to have his company. One cannot acquire a good character without a pure heart.'

Someone has said, 'One should protect his character all the time as it is the basis of his personality.' If one believes that he does not have good qualities and therefore cannot be wrong, then he is mistaken. This is his weakness. It is said that those who know their potential accurately should apply it with patience and show courage. As their attitude is pure, they will definitely gain energy to succeed.

So build your character with confidence, and make it pure and humble. If you have pure thoughts and a sound character, then you will stand tall in society. People will bow to you. Character is not something artificial that can be sold with a pleasant packaging. It is internal power that has to be generated by oneself.

Believe yourself, know yourself

A saint once said, 'Never trust others – Trust only yourself and your work. Being dependent on others puts you in trouble, while self-confidence is the real success.'

There is no greater power and truth than believing in yourself. The.moment we realize our true potential, we stop feeling anxious. Each step should be taken with confidence. We should estimate our true potential before beginning a task, it will help us accomplish it efficiently. If we are not sure of doing something, we should practice it beforehand. Dale Carnegie said, 'You should do what you don't like doing –

This will help your confidence grow, and take you towards the path of confidence'. Orison Swett Marden said, 'Each of us have immense potential inside – we can't even imagine how much inner-power we have. If we take an X-Ray of our inner self (self acknowledgement and self-realizing), we will be able to detect our talent, secret powers. It can take us to great heights, and help you rise above the level of the ordinary man and woman.'

A Unani thinker Sukarat engraved the following words on a wall, 'Know Yourself.' He knew that it is the key to success, both of the body and mind. People do not know their true potential, and most never try to explore it. But one can transform his life after gaining awareness. Orison Swett Marden wrote, 'When I came to know that this world needs me, I felt that I have the personality in me which is stronger than my outer appearance. This school was not a school for me but became a battleground where I have to fight every challenge to win it.' Russian writer Maxim Gorki also wrote 'Believe that you are the most essential person on this planet.'

We should take up every task with confidence. Those who quit do so because they are unaware of their worth. Emerson wrote, 'Those who depend on others are filled with grief, regret and disappointment, and fail to accomplish their task. These people make lame excuses and ultimately blame others for their own faults. But I ask them why they don't know their true potential, why don't they learn from this world? All the talents are present inside us and we need to nurture them. You haven't applied them in your life, and thus feel inferior to others. You waste your time worrying about other's success, but do not get inspired, or learn, from them. Why not? It is possible to succeed if you have the qualities of a successful man, but you will have to recognize them inside you first.'

Knowing yourself means knowing your potential and energy, and growing your confidence. It is said, 'Give someone a fish, and you feed him for a day. But teach him to fish, and you feed him for his whole life'. Frank Crain said, 'The mentors who guide their students towards self-discovery and self-awareness are truly great.' One identifies himself as successful, and grow accordingly with time. As he uses his talent, he nurtures it with practice. It is important to have faith in your talents in order to succeed in life. Your life will be decorated and fueled by your thoughts. One should remember that there is no point in succeeding without confidence. Do not think that you cannot do a particular task. If negativity enters your mind, then you can never accomplish it and hence cannot progress in life. Those who start confidently and hope to win end up succeeding. A thinker said, 'Lack of confidence is the real cause of failure. They are weak who do not believe in themselves, although they have enough potential inside to win.' Many courageous people have succeeded due to confidence and we can learn from them. Lord Tennyson said, 'Self-confidence, self-awareness and self control can make your life complete.'

Know your inner potential

Kaka Sahib Kalelkar, a follower of Gandhi, was questioned by a foreigner 'How could Gandhi impact society?' Kaka said, 'He had patience and a direct approach to society. He was firm in his decisions and spent all his life helping others.' This is the secret of being great, but it is possible only through confidence. Someone said, 'Even the toughest path becomes simple by confidence.' Lack of confidence is the reason for our failures. Those who do not trust themselves are weak and incapable.

There was a king whose Military Chief was very intelligent. One day, he asked his military chief, 'Which is the best weapon?' The Chief replied, 'The best weapon is confidence.' The king wanted proof. One day, they were coming back from the river after taking a bath. The street was narrow, and they met a mad elephant on the way. The chief threw his pot at the elephant's head, and it fell down. The king was scared, but the chief said, 'I did it because I had confidence.' And the king replied 'You are right, one can win a battle with confidence alone.'

Whatever challenges we face in life, we should have the confidence to succeed. Where there is confidence, there is potential to succeed. When one is doubtful, he never prepares well and does not attempt properly, and ultimately fails. A saying goes as, 'The one who believes, succeeds in life. Even God does not help the person who is not confident.' You need to trust yourself and believe in yourself – and you will surely succeed. Napoleon Bonaparte was a 'small' man in height, and no one could believe that he would one day take on the whole world. But Napoleon surprised everyone with his confidence and efforts. There are many people who have performed miracles with their confidence. Abraham Lincoln became the president of the USA, people crossed major oceans and climbed the loftiest mountain, and mankind even reached the moon. Pierre discovered the North Pole, a feat impossible to achieve without confidence. His companions opposed him and refused to move ahead, but he continued and succeeded. It is said, 'A confident person can make the impossible possible.'

Those who do not have faith in their own potential are unaware of their real worth. One should never think that he cannot succeed, as this doubt will stop us from trying, and, ultimately, from succeeding. Keep away your doubts and start to change your life.

Orison Swett Marden said, 'Confidence has immense power. One can overcome every obstacle in life.' Emerson said, 'Believe in yourself, this is an unbreakable string to connect your heart and soul.'

A thinker said, 'One cannot recover until he believes in the doctor and medicine. The real treatment lies in your inner belief.' It is the secret of success – believing in one's own self and making the necessary effort to win. So, one should trust his abilities in order to succeed in life. Swami Vivekananda said, 'There is no better friend than self confidence. It is the first step to success.'

❑

5

GOAL SETTING

- *Dedication towards goal*
- *Goal for every task*
- *Don't act without thinking*
- *It is necessary to inculcate the principles of success*
- *If and but*
- *The self-dependent person never feels depressed*
- *Identity of a true friend*
- *Why is discipline necessary?*
- *Time management and success*

Dedication towards goal

This story is from the epic *Mahabharat.* An insect was very worried. It laid its eggs on the battle ground, but was scared of them being trampled. It prayed to God for help and suddenly, a bell from an elephant's back fell down and covered the pit containing the eggs. When the war was over, somebody picked up the bell. The insects were safe and flew away. The insect thanked God. This story was enjoyed by students of saint Shamik. One student asked him, 'Lord, would God take our responsibility? Would he save us too? Shamik replied, 'My dear, where God stops, we have to begin. He made us capable of accomplishing our tasks and thus we can do it ourselves.' We tend to forget our own duties and responsibilities. Shamik said, 'God has done His job: Now, we have to do ours.'

We all have goals in life, but we are afraid to achieve them. We make excuses, are careless and delay the task. Whether it is education, competition, games or exams, etc., those who fully depend on God and do not do anything themselves cannot perform well. Even God does not help them. Those who do not study and pray to God for passing the exams, they are not heard by Him. You have to write the answers - otherwise, how will God help you? As you write, you will score. You have to work hard, and you will be rewarded accordingly.

It has been said in the Ramcharitramanas –

'Karm pradhan vishwa kari rakha, jo jas karai so tas fal chakha'.

Napoleon said, 'One should do his job himself to make it successful and beautiful.'

Orison Swett Marden writes 'God has sent everyone to this world for some purpose. All of you are here for some duty, and you should perform it well. Throw away all your doubts and think about your benefit. Nurture good thoughts in your mind and start working hard. This will bring confidence and passion to your work, and you will be able to accomplish all tasks successfully.'

We are discussing goals. If one wants to succeed, he must have specific goals in life. One cannot succeed without goals. Shakespeare said, 'If you have decided to finish a task, never quit it because of petty reasons. Believe from the beginning that you will face problems, and that you will need to overcome them. But stepping back from them is cowardice.' Vinobha Bhave said, 'Begin the task and if you have begun it, finish it.'

Life offers us many challenges and there is no person on earth who does not have to face them. Every task is a challenge. There is no smooth road. Hence, we do not have to worry about them; we just have to finish our job. Those who fight challenges succeed in life and achieve their goals. A thinker asked Abraham Lincoln, 'If you want popularity, you should learn grammar.' Lincoln started learning grammar since that day. He faced many problems, he was very poor and could not afford electricity in his house. He studied under the light of woods and ashes. Finally, he succeeded, and, indeed, went on to become the president of USA. Gandhiji said, 'Do not think about the results, do your work. Work without expectations.' This is also written in the Gita. The one who does not work falls down very badly. One who does not expect receives more from his work. Passionate people finish their jobs in time and never step back. One who is passionate about his goals can never be defeated.

Goal for every task

There was a king who was indecisive and acted upon others' advice. He wondered how to recognize opportunities in life. He asked this question publicly and all thinkers, poets, astrologers, pundits, etc., came forward with their opinions. One said, 'We should ask an astrologer'. Others suggested the advice of old men. But the king was confused and did not get the answer he was looking for. One day, he saw a saint in an ashram and decided to ask him. The saint was ploughing his field. The king greeted him and asked his question, but the saint remained silent. He went to the saint the next day, but found the same response. He visited many days continuously and came back without an answer. One day, he asked, 'Why do you not give me a reply?' The saint replied, 'I answered you the very first day. The best time to begin a task is NOW! This means that every moment of your life is 'opportune'. You have to utilise your time and begin the work. You should not wait for the right time.' The king got his answer.

We should have one aim within us and make sincere efforts to attain it. How can we reach our destination if we do not even start? People think of beginning a task on the 'perfect time' and wait for others' help. The 'perfect time' never comes and our task remains incomplete.

Thinkers believe that we should not wait for ideal circumstances but make the present circumstances ideal. It is upto us to reach our goals. Turning circumstances in your favour is the ability to grab opportunity. Napoleon said, 'Give me one chance and see the miracles.' Those who utilize their opportunities move ahead in life.

Benjamin Disraeli said, 'Man's success lies in making the best of every situation.' Benjamin Franklin said, 'There were some labourers constructing a house near my office. I noticed that they were always happy. They radiated a certain sparkle due to their positive energy. They were not upset by climatic variations, financial ups & downs, etc.' He met them and asked them the secret of being happy. One labourer replied, 'It is too simple. My wife is very humble and motivates me whenever I leave for my job and welcomes me whenever I return home. She offers me a cup of tea and treats me well. This is the secret of my happiness.' These kinds of people are very passionate about their job, and down-to-earth at the same time. They utilize their opportunities to excel in life.

Everyone does not get the opportunity, rather, they cannot identify it. Hence, one should finish a task at the earliest time and opportunity to do so. No one knows if we will get the same chance the next day, or not. Never wait for a 'perfect time'. A Unani playwright said, 'Opportunity does not help those who do not help himself.' One has to be dedicated to finish a task – this is the secret of great men's success. Dedication and opportunity go hand in hand. According to the Irish philosopher Edmund Burke, 'Our image is our real booster. It helps us to identify our goals and compels us to move ahead in life. It not only enables us to touch great heights, but also taste the depths and range of success.' Therefore, one should avail every opportunity that comes one's way and never think about obstructions and road blocks. Life examines us from many angles and tests, and rewards us on passing it. You might have got many chances to study, play, appear for interview, etc., but they all demanded hard work. The same opportunity never knocks twice – so you have to grab it as soon as it comes. Many students say that they will clear the exam next time but what can be the reason of their failure? You may not be able to appear the next time or might not clear it. Then, who will help you out? Shakespeare, said 'Man's behavior is like a volcano; If you can control it, you can reach the final level of success.'

Don't act without thinking

There is a Hindi proverb, *'Bina vichare jo kare, so pachhe pachtaye,'* which means 'If you act without due consideration or thought, you will regret it later.' It is necessary to think intelligently before performing any action; otherwise the outcome could be dangerous or negative. A king and his troops were passing through Rajasthan. They were tired from their journey and decided to take rest under tree. The troops saw bunches of fruits in the tree and wanted to taste them. The wise leader stopped them and said, 'If the fruits had been worth eating, then other troops passing before us would have already eaten them up.' Later, they came to know that the fruits were, indeed, poisoned. The leader said, 'One should think twice before acting... because one has to live with the consequences for the rest of one's life.'

Confucius said, 'Learning without thinking is a waste of energy, and thinking without education is even more harmful.' Many people initiate a task without giving it any thought, and put themselves in trouble. Instant decision can create more problems than it solves.

There are many stories from our ancient times which teach us the virtues and benefits of a decisive mind. King Sagar lost 60,000 children after being cursed by Guru Kapil. King Dashrath was cursed to be isolated from his child on killing Shravan Kumar. Both kings paid heavily for their spontaneous actions. So, a task should be done after careful consideration. A thinker said, 'Great ideas become great when they see the light of reality.' Thought is first created in mind and then it is processed. But one has to think about the outcome of the process. Sadly, people do not follow this step and try to find short-cuts, and finally fail. People want instant success without thinking about the pros and cons. People do not want to spend time in learning but want to gain results as soon as possible. The result is failure. There is an English proverb, 'Think before you leap'. Hence, one should remember to think and work patiently. Expecting results in a hurry is like choosing the path of failure. It is necessary to lay the foundation stones for any task before beginning it, and it needs immense patience and tolerance to be executed. One can only succeed by taking fair decisions based on proper thoughts in order to succeed. People who live a life of fantasy end up losing their potential. A thinker writes 'People tend to work without belief and feel disappointed on failing. Incomplete beliefs never reap complete results.' The reason behind one's failure lies in one's hurriedness, half-hearted attempts and impatience. People think that hurried nature is a quality to cherish – this misconception hurts them as a result. They do not want to work consistently and look for magic solutions. They do not want to spend time in learning and do not practice their work. They want to be rich overnight without making efforts. These people can never succeed in life.

Chanakya wanted Chandragupta Maurya to become the emperor of the country, but he was facing obstacles. So, both of them stayed in disguise in a village with an old lady. She had a grandchild who approached her and asked for a meal. The lady served him food and he started eating, but he burned his tongue because the food was hot. The lady said, 'You are like Chandragupta who starts fighting suddenly. You should have waited for it to cool down before eating. If Chandragupta plans his wars with due consideration and strategy, he too can win.' Chandragupta understood his mistake and planned his future moves with care and precision, and eventually became the emperor of the country. One should think before acting.

It is necessary to inculcate the principles of success

This is a competitive world and there is no field where there is no competition. The one who supersedes every problem is the best. Earlier, people believed that success meant getting comforts of life. But today, the meaning has changed. People want more than comforts and they want it instantly but they are still not satisfied. They are hungry for more money, promotions, contracts, success, etc. However, when one does not get everything that one desires, he feels depressed. His mind breaks down, and he contacts diseases like diabetes, heart disease, BP, etc. It is common to observe these diseases in people in the age group of 35 and more, and the reason is dissatisfaction.

The competition today has multiplied to a great extent. Employers get their employees to work for upto 18 hours a day sometimes, and they are buried under a heavy load of work. Man can work these hours up to a certain extent very easily, but loses his capacity in the long run. His graph falls down, which affects his performance. But the company wants profits at the same level, and he gets thrown out of his job. It is a vicious cycle. People used to trust and respect experienced employees, but today most companies do not care about such people. They only want profit – at any cost. The real meaning of success is drastically changing. The one who is fetching the highest salary is the most successful and gets promotions. Likewise, there are different parameters of success in the fields of business, sports or education. People believe that students scoring more marks are successful and compel their children to score higher and higher – sometimes even above 98%. Students receive gold medals in their exams but it doesn't guarantee success later on in life. I know an IAS officer who always came first in life, but could not prove himself a good administrator in his career. His juniors got promoted ahead of him, and he retired at the same designation level that he had joined. Hence, being a bookworm or being ranked first does not guarantee your success in life.

One has to know the secrets of success in life based up on the field he chooses. You have to adapt to the situation. A thinker has written, 'Success is not the collection of parameters or knowledge. These are just the parts of success.' A knowledgeable person can be unsuccessful, while one without knowledge can succeed. Failure indicates that the necessary effort has not been made to succeed. We lack the technique to succeed and one cannot dream of success without this. So, success is a technique that adapts knowledge to the situation and circumstance.

The values of our life are changing rapidly, and changing our behavior and routine as well. People expect changes in traditional thoughts and cultural values. There is a tremendous change in routine habits, tastes and preferences, and the change of values is not surprising. The principles of success will also change due to change in the behavior of a human being. We need to understand these things and adopt them wisely. Someone has rightly said, 'Fresh thought and planning are the basis of progress and success. These apply in both physical and spiritual life. The evolution of new trends and behaviors is a result of this sea-change in human attitude. These principles can be applied to any area of life.' Therefore, one can succeed only by adapting oneself according to the circumstances and this should be our goal.

If and but

Many people try to make excuses by saying 'if' and 'but' before starting any task. They keep on saying, 'If I had money….. if someone could have helped me…. if I knew some politician….' etc. The excuses are endless and such people cannot begin any task with conviction. Even if they do, they feel they cannot complete it, and eventually, that's exactly how things turn out. They are more interested in finding excuses than putting in their efforts. They cannot take charge or responsibility for any job. No one helps them because they do not deserve it. A thinker says, 'Be positive and know your potential. Know yourself and win this world.' Merry T Russell wrote 'People do not succeed because they do not know themselves properly. So be positive and grow your potential. Say with conviction – I am a peaceful soul – and you will truly become so. If you think that you are restless, you will become so. Everyone changes himself. When you get up in the morning, say to yourself 'I have the potential to become what I like to be. I have decided to be happy, passionate, calm and patient.' Once you say this to your subconscious mind, it will help you achieve this goal. But if you say that you are exhausted, you hate yourself and you are a failure, then you will certainly destroy your self-image. Hence, never think negatively about what you do or what you want to happen in your life.'

Try to be an optimistic person and remember that only an optimistic person reaps the fruits of success. It is true that those who succeed in life are the ones who had desired to get the best. Hence, wish for the best and not the worst because you are going to get what you have desired.

A thinker has said, 'Life can be a satisfactory experience if you are aware of your similarities and dissimilarities with other creatures. Live on the principles of life and nature and accept their worth. Nurture them because every successful person has brought peace into his life by following these principles.' In fact, God gives us peace, He is the judge of our efforts. But unfortunately, we do not value these rules.

Only positive thought can help us reach our goals. When you think positively, you adopt a positive approach in life and find solutions to all your problems. You start filtering your habits positively, as they pass through your subconscious mind. If you can control your thoughts, then you can control your life too. You can throw away all the negative thoughts in your life. It makes your soul so light that trouble can never reach your level of success.

Positive people are also depressed sometimes – after all, we are all human. You will agree that all human beings are controlled by their emotions. Strong emotions or thoughts can make a person hesitant and react accordingly. It does not mean that you should give up in these hard times. Positive thinkers increase their capacity at this time and overcome all such circumstances with their sheer efforts. Hence, be a positive thinker and direct your life through a proper channel. If you inculcate a habit of saying 'Yes,' then you will feel that you are automatically energized for your tasks and duties in life. This will go on to create miracles in your life.

The self-dependent person never feels depressed

A self-dependent person never feels depressed. Once, villagers were leaving their village because of a flood and were moving to a different place with all their valuables. Among them was a person who did not have any possession, and had a smile on his face. Someone asked him, 'Everyone is crying and worrying for their future while you are looking happy and peaceful. Aren't you scared of your future? And where is your luggage?' The man replied, 'I have everything with me in the form of confidence. I have belief that a better future lies ahead, because I know I can get back all that I have lost. So why do I need to cry when I can earn it back again?'

A self-sufficient person knows his potential and never fails in life. Self-belief teaches us to acknowledge our potential and grow in life. These people move ahead with the conviction to overcome all odds and succeed, and, naturally, these people have a glow on their face – like the villager who is confident that he will find a solution to his problems, even though he is forced to live in a forest. These people can achieve the toughest goals with the simplest resources. They have the passion to achieve their goals and they do it.

Identity of a true friend

Arthur Schopenhauer was a visionary who wanted to discuss his thoughts with his friends. He wanted that they should share their experiences amongst one another and learn from them. But all his friends were corrupt, dishonest and greedy, and he felt very sad about it. It was his opinion that people were forgetting their true values in life, and hence he made no friends in life. But he found a true friend in a dog and he used to call him 'Soul.' Schopenhauer wrote about his life's troubles, 'I have spent all my life in isolation without a friend. When I think about it, I feel disappointed. Do you know what I prayed to God for? I used to ask Him for a true friend but God didn't listen to my prayers. I might be wrong, or may have lacked the art of making friends, but it is not justice. The reason behind my isolation is that I found no humanity left in anyone. They deserted me when I needed them the most. Every one duped me and disappointed me. I could not share my sorrow with others and no one came forward in my time of true need, like a true friend would.'

In reality, friendship is a mutual relationship where both persons have to express happiness in each other's company. It is important to maintain a balance between the two and they should not be selfish. When the balance is lost, the friendship ends and the one responsible for the break loses a good friend. Disraeli says, 'Friendship is a blessing from God and essential for human survival.'

When we think about Schopenhauer, we know that it is really difficult to find a true friend in life. If one gets a real friend, he should remember to strike a balance between his friendship and professional life. One should also agree to Benjamin Franklin's words, 'There are only three real kinds of friends – old wife, old dog and saved money. So are we to spend our lives without friends? No, that is wrong. But one should test the friend before trusting him.' Poet Ramdhari Singh Dinkar has written in his book *Rashmirathi*, 'Friendship is a valuable jewel and it cannot be priced in terms of money.' The *Mahabharata* says that Karan gave up his life for friendship.

Who is a true friend? Many visionaries and thinkers have written about it. Rahim says:

'mathat mathat makhan rahe, dahi mahi bilgaye,
rahiman soi meet hai, bhir pari thahraye.'

English philosopher Francis Bacon said, 'A true friend multiplies the charm in your life.' Happiness and anxiety represent the presence of a friend and foe respectively. Chinese thinker Confucius said, 'Do not make a friend who is not better than you.' It also applies in all aspects of life. But you have to make friends in every walk of life – be it school, college, office, business, etc, and therefore you must understand the true meaning of a 'friend', and the true value of friendship. One should also know the key to make a friend. It is said 'A friend in need is a friend indeed.'

According to Hitopdesha:

Parokshe karyahantaram pratakshya priyavadinam,
Varjyatadrisham mitra vishkumbhama payomutvam.

Those who speak sweet in front of you but bite behind your back are no different from toxic elements.

In the Ramayana, sage Valmiki says:

Rajtam va suvarnava shubhanyabharnani cha,
avibhaktani sadhunamvagachcanti sadhavah.

Good friends do not see any difference between their friends, and jewels.

Socrates said, 'Never be in a hurry to make friends, but maintain the friendship till the end.'

Hence, make friends carefully, and keep the friendship forever.

Why is discipline necessary?

We greet the sun every morning and it sets every evening, only to rise again the following morning. Likewise, one season follows another. This cycle has been happening for billions of years and will continue the same way. Indeed, nature follows a discipline – a balanced discipline, which we, too, can apply in our lives. We know that when there is imbalance in nature, it causes destruction in the form of storms, earthquakes, heavy rains, floods, etc. Nature advices us to be disciplined and often warns us to adhere to a discipline. But how often do we think about it? Do we know how much disciplined we are ourselves? The answers to these questions could surprise and even shock us. We would then understand that we alone – and noone else – are responsible for our failures.

What are the roots of hate and loathing in society? We want a good job, a good business and a good companion. But do we make efforts for it? No, not really. If we think deeply, then we will see that there are three central aspects of life – discipline, values and balance. A thinker said, 'Discipline is categorized as internal and external. Internal discipline is more important because until you control yourself, you cannot control the outside world. Disciplined flow of water is a good example and teaches us valuable lessons. But when the flow breaks, it creates disaster and spoils the life of thousands of people. So, in this way, nature warns us every moment to be disciplined.'

When we live a life of indiscipline, we block our paths to success. On the other hand, if we follow discipline in our life, it paves the way for success. People generally feel that they are being forced to work under discipline, but they do not know that this is important for their own good. It is not a restriction but freedom to achieve more in life.

When we are living a disciplined life, we see positive changes coming on in our lives and in ourselves. We advance towards our success and build our character as per our requirement to gain victory. Our character governs our lives and represents our true personality. If we are not disciplined, it will reflect in our personality, and we will end up worthless.

Lilli Allen has exemplified and defined character as, 'It is good to know the meaning of character. We should be clear about this. Shouting our loud by ego, self-importance and a swollen pride is not a sign of good character. Befooling others and speaking without thinking is again not character. A sound character needs no added colour or flamboyance, and can be observed naturally. A person does not need to make any extra effort to present his character to others - it is visible through his work.' One's character should not be forcibly imposed or affected by insults, laziness, etc. These habits create havoc and miseries in life. Until a person applies purity and generosity in his life, he cannot attain a gentle and decent character. He will not understand the value of self-respect and never acquire the qualities of a successful man. Hence, everyone should maintain his self-respect and not act like lunatics. James Allen says, 'Feeling inferior to others is the worst kind of thought to possess, and is akin to committing suicide. These people become impotent and destroy their lives completely.'

Therefore, it is very important to follow discipline in life. We can build a sound character through it and hone our daily life to soar the dizzying heights of success.

Time management and success

According to Dr Radhakrishnan, Indian culture was defined and differentiated by its non-violence, and its abstaining from audacity and violence. Mahavira's non-violence is based on kindness towards every creature on this earth. When we talk of Gandhiji and non-violence, we remember the following words of Einstein, 'The coming generations would not be able to believe that there was a person like Gandhi on this earth.' While English author H G Wales believed in the concept of non-violence due to doubts in his character, Gandhiji had a completely (100%, and not in parts) non-violent attitude.

Chakravarti Rajagopalachari (Rajaji), the Governor of Bengal, was in Calcutta to meet Gandhiji. There was a girl busy peeling peas in the conference room. Gandhiji said, 'Look at this girl attacking her work.' But the girl was concentrating deeply in her work, and every one thought, how could she be attacking? Then Gandhiji indicated the peas that were rammed under the shoes on the floor, and some parts that were wasted around the rim of the bowl. Everyone understood. According to Gandhiji, carelessness was equivalent to attacking. He used to say, "Beauty is truth. If some eatable is destroyed, then it is an attack to truth. Time is also a truth and one should be punctual. Purity is a divine form of truth and non-violence can never break this rule. Thus, every natural product is beneficial for a human being. If these are being disturbed and destroyed, then you must consider it as violence.'

The types of violence discussed above are considered to be true by thinkers and visionaries alike. They warn us to safeguard against them. The most important of all is killing time; we cannot get it back. One can have everything in life except time. Yet we waste time playing cards and sleeping!

Time is one of the most precious things in life. The one who loses time regrets it his entire life. Ancient philosophers preached about utilizing the time in the best possible way. 'You should get up before the sun rises even if you have no tasks to do. This way, you will get rid of the habit of laziness and nurture your mind well. Never forget that you will waste your whole day if you sleep till late morning.'

This is time management. It helps us make better use of our life. Those who managed their time well and spent it wisely and, mostly, ended up becoming popular and successful in society. The list is endless: Abraham Lincoln, Henry Ford, Newton, Einstein, Julius Caeser, etc.

It is said that those who can 'catches time' always has enough of it. Somebody asked Alexander the great, 'How could you conquer the world?' Alexander replied, 'The reason behind my success is my dedication and proper planning.' Those who do not utilize their time to plan their life remain unsuccessful.

One should understand the value of time and he can hone his skills by time management. Someone has rightly said, 'Time is the greatest of all, greater than God. One can call God with prayers, but not time.' Therefore, it is important to utilize time wisely. Shakespeare said, 'If you destroy time, it will destroy you.'

❑

6

LIFE BEHAVIOR

- *First, learn to behave*
- *Be patient*
- *What is patience?*
- *Gre et but carefully*
- *Are you an emotional fool?*
- *Be careful about appraisal and criticism!*
- *Never criticise others*
- *Never boast of your achievements*
- *Think before you speak*
- *Words are sharper than sword*
- *Be careful about friends*
- *Who should be our friend?*
- *It's our habit, but...*
- *Make your habits your servant, not master*
- *Petty is crucial*

First, learn to behave

American president Abraham Lincoln, during his student life, used to work as a labourer to pay his school fees. He once joined an office as a salesman and collected an extra dollar from a customer in a hurry. Later, when he found out the mistake after calculating, he went to his customer's house and apologized for his mistake while returning the dollar. He returned it late at night, but, made a good friend. It is important to have a sound character. The more humble a person is, the more popular he becomes. He will be respected well in the society, and be listened to and helped by everyone. Speaking sweetly, helping others and guiding them do not harm you in any way. We should be alert about our behavior, and behave according to the situation. Some people behave superficially in different environments.

The famous German poet Goethe said, 'Man's behavior is a reflection of his personality.' How true! We can understand the emotions of a person through his expressions. If we are not behaving well, we can see the disapproval and dissatisfaction in others' eyes. His expressions will clearly communicate his desire to stay separate from others. English author Dr. Samuel Johnson wrote 'A gentle behavior deserves to enter into everyone's heart.' One day, a person asked him, 'I live a life of honesty but no one appreciates me.' And he replied 'It is good to be honest but you need to be gentle in your behavior. Then you will be appreciated for ever, and be loved by all.' Emerson said, 'Good behavior is attained by sacrificing petty arguments'. These days, we often forget to thank others and do not feel sorry for others in difficulty. These things affect us in the long run, and applying these qualities result in positive outcomes.

The Bible says that you must treat others as you would like to be treated yourself. We should not be partial in our behavior, and should remain consistent in form and attitude. Every person possesses self-respect, and one who understands, remembers and respects it, is a real gentleman. Even a little arrogance can be dangerous. We should, therefore, take extreme caution while dealing with others. The importance of behavior can be easily understood from the Hitopdesha:

No Kaschitkasyachinmitram na kaschitkasyachidripu,
Vyavharen mitrani jayante ripvashtha.

No one is friend or a foe, but becomes so by our behavior. Thus, behavior is called the backbone of one's perso[illegible] is said that words are powerful and crucial. They are like knives – they can penetrate the heart and really hurt. Words can make or break relationships. So, one should be gentle and soft-spoken in order to build relations. Charles Dickens had a soft speech that was very endearing and popular, and Goethe was well known for his humility and modest behavior. Napoleon's wife was a very gentle lady.

We sometimes feel hurt from others' behavior, but we need to learn actually from them. It tells us that we should not behave in a similar (rude) way to others, as others would feel bad. We behave in an ill-mannered way occasionally, but this is our loss, because by that, we can lose even good friends and strong relationships. A G Gardner said, 'As bad behavior affects negatively, similarly, good behavior also leaves its long-lasting impact.' So, it is better to behave in a proper manner.

We can develop politeness only by practicing. It is a good quality to speak softly and try to understand others' point of view. Rabindranath Tagore said, 'We are closer to greatness when we are polite.' Hence, we should be aware of this habit, inculcate it and analyze it regularly. Success truly depends upon our behavior and it is a necessary ingredient for one to make a positive impact in life.

Be patient

You might have heard the tale of a hen that used to lay golden eggs. The owner used to earn a handsome amount from the eggs, but one day he became greedy, and wanted all the money at one go. He lost his patience, and killed the hen, but got nothing except regrets. There were, obviously, no eggs inside. He lost his source of income, and the chance to have a bright future.

It is very important to be patient in performing daily tasks. Some people do not understand the value of patience, and end up losing because of their haste and hurry. When elders advice them, they do not hear. The world is full of talented people who have failed because they tried to apply shortcuts in life, and gained nothing in the end. They want to become rich overnight and get instant results, even if it meant resorting to unfair means. How long can they maintain their success? Trouble is bound to befall them.

Let us analyse ourselves and know what we really want to achieve in life, and what are the conditions that need to be fulfilled? Let us take the example of making tea. The water will take its own time to boil, you cannot hurry the process. Rice, pulses and grains will take their own specific time to be cooked. A child will grow gradually with time, and you cannot hurry their developmental process. A tree will bear fruits after a certain specific period. An aeroplane will also take its time to reach its destination and you will have to be patient. If you drive in a hurry, the outcome could be a fatal accident. Every job takes time. There is no shortcut to success. Learn from nature... even nature follows time.

Confucius said, 'Learning without thinking is a waste of energy and thinking without education is even more hurtful.' Many people begin a task without giving any thought to it, and invite trouble, naturally.

It is rightly said that the one who is not afraid of hard work and remains patient wins in life. Only the impatient follow shortcuts. Their success is an illusion and short lived. Thus, one should exercise patience in his work. Maharishi Valmiki wrote

Vyasane varthkrichhe va bhaye va jivitantage,
Vimreshanshach svaya budbyha dhritimannavisidati.

One who exercises patience in trouble, financial crisis and extreme situations never face difficulties in life. The Gita has explained the philosophy of working without expectations, and one should follow it heartfully. If you go against the concept, you will endanger your chances of success, and it will increase your mental anxiety. So, it is better to work honestly and wait for the results.

What is patience?

Saint Tukaram of Maharashtra used to donate all his money to the poor. As a result, there wasn't a single grain of food in his house and his wife said, 'Go and get some sugarcane from the field.' Tukaram went, but as was his nature, distributed all the sugarcane among the needy, and, as always, was left with one for himself. His wife got angry and beat him with the same sugarcane and it broke into two pieces. Tukaram said, 'It is good that you have split the cane in two... now we both can relish its taste.' His wife was ashamed.

Patience is a quality that all of us can use in our lives. In fact, we suggest others to be patient, but do not follow it ourselves. We start fighting while standing in long queues, but never stop suggesting others not to do so.

In reality, patience is the best quality of a person, but it takes enormous practice to nurture it. Somebody asked England's Prime Minister William Pitt, 'What is the biggest quality of a prime minister? He replied promptly, in one word, 'Patience'.

Many people do not care to inculcate the habit of practice in life. Students want to clear their exams by studying less, the youth today want to succeed overnight, businessmen want instant profits, the list is endless. We seem to want everything in life, without making efforts. Everyone wants to overtake others on the road to success, and do not want to wait at the red signals. I observed the same example when a person overtook me and then waited on red signal. I asked him 'What was the use of driving so fast, when both of us are finally stuck at the same red signal?'

A thinker said, 'Impatience is the sign of an imbalanced mind.' An impatient person wants to work hurriedly and needs instant results. He either ruins the assignment, or quits the task mid-way and loses his confidence. Gradually, people stop trusting him with responsibility, and he feels inferior to others. Ruskin said, 'Some succeed in every thing they do while others fail in the same things. The difference lies in patience. A patient person will win over the restless one.' You might have read the story of the rabbit and the tortoise in your childhood. The message is simple yet powerfully true – 'Slow and steady wins the race'.

If you read about thinkers, scientists, inventors and visionaries, you will discover how most of them were extremely patient people. In fact, they would never have become great without patience.

Sadly, today's youth seems to have forgotten all this, and is running blindly in the rat-race of life - where he has not even learnt to walk properly. Hence, it is absolutely necessary to be patient with others - it is a test of our personality. We have to meet many people everyday. Different characters have to be tackled differently.

The path of patience is the best, but also the most difficult. We can maintain the balance by being patient and it gives us the power to achieve more in life. Everyone is busy with his problems and wants to live peacefully. We should be satisfied with what we have, and feel happy about it. Boasting of our possessions is not a sign of success. It leaves a negative impact on others.

Greet but carefully

New Year is the season of wishing others and it is a good business season for card manufacturers and sellers. It's easy to wish friends, relatives or closed ones in this hectic life. One can find time for others at least once in a year. There is no denying that there are many greetings available in the market during the festive season. Moreover, you can also find appropriate cards for birthdays, anniversaries, success, promotions, etc. What can be a better option than greeting others in such a beautiful manner? People generally tend to greet others through cards, if not personally.

The way we greet others has changed, and today people are saying 'Hi' instead of 'Namaste.' This contains no love, affection or emotion. The world is changing very fast, but is also proceeding towards ruin. People living in flats do not know their neighbours and they do not even *want* to know about them. People are feeling jealous of each other. This is not a sign of our beautiful culture, but reflects the symptoms of a disease. Can we eliminate the differences between us? The best solution is that we should greet each other without selfishness and feel good about them. At least we will have one link, and feel good about it in our hearts. Andrew Carnegie said, 'The secret of happiness lies in giving it, and not asking for it.' We can multiply our happiness by sharing it. So, sending beautiful cards is a sign of gentle traditions.

We send greetings during festivals and the post office usually makes special arrangements for it. People send their cards in bulk amounts, which is commercialization. There are people who send printed cards where the address is printed on the envelope which, again, is commercialization. If you work hard, you can make your own greetings and send them with your personalized emotions. It will be appreciated tenfold more.

Be careful about choosing cards and read all the contents of the card before buying it. Hilarious cards can irritate others or they might consider it 'improper'. Never send cards with sexual images in it as it is not a good indicator of decency or personality. Your reader should take a personal interest in your cards and you must be able to explain your feelings genuinely through it. If you receive a card for an invitation, never forget to thank. Send your greetings in advance, so as to reach them in time.

You will receive many greetings and you should thank the sender for it. This sweet emotion links us together – and all of us are hungry for genuine emotions. Humanity teaches us to be sweet and affectionate to each other. People should help others in difficult times and behave properly. Never consider salutations like Namaste, Jai Ram, Assalam Aleikum, etc; to be too traditional or 'stuffy' to greet others with: If the situation demands it, and if it expresses the feelings of your heart accurately, then by all means use such greetings. This is the mark of our culture. Can we maintain peace and harmony with jealousy and acrimony?

Are you an emotional fool?

There was a saint who had many students. One of them died. The saint started crying inconsolably, and this surprised his other disciples. After all, he had taught his students about the importance of the soul (over the earthly body), but today he himself was crying over the body. Was not the soul eternal? Then why was he so much attached to the body? They asked him, 'Guru-ji, why are you crying?' The saint replied, 'I cannot answer your question'. But the students urged him to answer them and he replied, 'I know the soul is eternal, but I cannot help myself.' The students asked again, 'Are you crying for the dead body?' The guru said 'My soul is crying, and not me. So, what should I do now?' The students were confused and could not understand the concept. They asked again, 'Are you crying for the body?' The saint replied, 'Maybe; My student was very loving to me and I will not be able to see him again.' The students reminded him of spirituality and tried to stop him from crying, but the saint replied, 'I am in an illusion. Life is so strange that I cannot decide what should be done.' The students were quiet for some days, but found that their guru was still upset, and asked again. Now, the saint replied, 'If someone is unhappy, let him find peace. The more you ask, the more depressed he will be. One needs a normal situation to become normal. I know that it is not necessary to cry on his death, but had I not cried, people would have said that I am a hard-hearted man who did not cry on his student's death. So, it is essential to maintain a balance between normal and special conditions. I felt satisfied after crying and it released some load from my mind. The soul is eternal while the body is destructible, but we cannot escape its earthly callings completely.'

We are losing emotional content from society and becoming self-centered. There is no scope for release of emotions these days, and generous and sincere people are considered 'fools'. When children go abroad and leave behind their old parents, they say, 'Why are you crying? I am going to build my career. You have lived your life, now let me live mine.

I will keep sending money to you to enjoy the luxuries of life. What more do you want from me?' But he can never pay for the time he is spending away from his family. The old will definitely die one day, but the value of their life is not being understood by youth. Can you compare emotions with money?

This attitude is growing in our society. Do children in joint families respect their elders? We are more concerned about our friends, colleagues and professional life but not our parents. The truth is that we are losing emotions with time and living a hollow life. Can we live without emotions? It is a part of life and we cannot sustain life without them.

Actually, there are two categories of people in our society i.e. those who are becoming emotionless and destroying their life by living in a vacuum, and those who are living a life of extreme, unbalanced emotions. Neither of these two states is good for anyone, and we need to maintain a balance between the two. Dominance of either state can be harmful.

Be careful about appraisal and criticism!

There is an ancient story about a boy named Atul who approached Revat, Sariputra and Anand, the disciples of Lord Buddha to learn from them. But after a few days, he approached Lord Buddha and said, 'I went to Revat, but he didn't respond to me. Sariputra taught me religion but I could not understand him, and Anand spoke very little. Thus, I am here to learn from you.' Buddha heard him, smiled and said, 'Atul, people have been appreciating and criticising both the mute and the talkative ones since ancient times. People also appreciate and criticise the sun, stars and nature. So, criticism or appreciation of this nature is worthless. Only an intelligent man's appraisal or criticism is worth thinking about.

We face both criticism and appreciation in our lives. Some people try to manipulate our minds, while others only like to criticize. They are experts in insulting even geniuses. But the truth is that none of them is important for us. Actually, these words have lost their worth. People love characterless politicians and criticise honest men. It is all happening around us.

These issues and questions are quite important for us, and especially so for the next generation, which has to face the consequences themselves later. This is the truth. No generation will accept this cruelty.

If we measure appreciation and criticism, we will realize that it acts like a guide for us and teaches us the value of life at every step. We are inspired by an appraisal and feel respected. But sometimes, we are carried away by emotions and seek more appreciation with fewer efforts. Thus, we tend to expect more and feel depressed on not acquiring it. Politics introduced diplomacy to society. People started expecting more and quibbled to seniors. Politicians followed tactfulness after independence and gained sympathy. Our society is going down due to these corrupt politicians. We are doing nothing about it, and hope that our new generation can handle it. A Roman visionary said 400 years ago, 'You can gain an understanding about someone's personality by his reaction to appreciation.' This is true and valid up to a great extent. You will have to clean the gutter of this dirty society and keep it clean. Corruption has increased because of diplomacy, and its misuse can be severely harmful to all of us in the future.

Similarly, a critic should be heard carefully, for we can learn a lot from him. However, when a person criticises you like a foe, you should beware of him. People criticise in the parliament when in opposition, but forget that they too will be criticised tomorrow. They play with criticism, and it turns around to attack them back. Therefore, this is a mis-step. Kabir said;

'nindak niyre rakhiye, angan kuti chavay.'

It means that you can never gain from a critic if you treat him like your enemy. Conversely, a critic's real role is to bring you back to the right path. Hence, it is said

'Bina pani sabun bina, nirmal kare subhaye.'

Hence, we will have to understand a critic's point of view intelligently, and utilise them constructively. The one who is alarmed by appreciation and refined by criticism can become successful. This attitude will purify our society. Should we not do something about it?

Never criticise others

We generally blame others and are more interested in finding others' faults. Finding others' faults is itself a fault and feeling joyous criticizing others is a crime. If we do some self-analysis, we will realize that we are wasting previous time and opportunity in knocking others down, rather than nurturing our talents. This can be done by changing our attitude. Adopt the habit to look for other's good qualities, as everyone has some quality - and so do you. Thinkers say that we should make a list of our friends, relatives and acquaintances, and write down their qualities – and you will find some qualities that they possess but you do not. This will make you start appreciating them.

Some people boast about their own qualities all the time, and do not listen to others. This is a bad habit. Remember: If you do not listen to others, they will not listen to you. Let both of you speak intermittently. Be sweet and soft-spoken and listen intently and patiently. Ask about the other person's health and his family, and let him feel at home with you. He will experience calm in the relationship, and respond to you positively.

There was a saint praying in the forest. A king and his soldiers were hunting there and the king got separated from them. A soldier asked the saint, 'Have you seen the king?' The saint remained quiet and prayed to God. Then, the chief appeared and asked 'Lord, did our king come here?' The saint continued to be quiet and busy in his prayer. The soldiers got irritated and went away. After some time, the king appeared and said, 'I apologize for disturbing you, but please tell if my soldiers were here.' The saint replied, 'Yes, they were here.' King asked how he knew, since he was sitting with his eyes closed. The saint replied that he came to know about it through their conversation.

Our identity is reflected by our words and it paints our character accordingly. This is a habit that can be polished by practice, and we can gain much through it. Ego, anger, jealousy and impatience are the enemies of gentle behavior. The one who wants to succeed must throw away ego, jealousy, impatience and anger. You should behave and speak in such a way that your mannerism and words impresses and pleases others.

Many people do not give this any importance and forget that even a needle could be more important than a sword. Everything has its own importance. A small ant can kill a giant elephant. A matchstick can burn a whole town. A small mistake can take the shape of a disaster.

Thus, those who think before speaking and act wisely gain success in life. But when you speak with a forked tongue, you lose your relations and people start avoiding you.

Therefore, it is not good on your part to speak ill of others and behave rudely with them. You should know your potential and emerge as a new person. You will then keep on progressing day after day.

Never boast of your achievements

There was a thirsty person who went to the ocean to quench his thirst. He gulped the water, then vomited it out immediately. He thought that the ocean is useless for human being and that the river is much better because it can quench one's thirst. He heard someone say, 'You thought correctly. The river generously and dutifully distributes all its water and healing energy before entering the ocean. It waters the fields and feeds the trees and animals, but doesn't have an ego- Whereas the ocean boasts of its size and strength, but does not know that there is no use of just being huge. The river is happy to help others while the ocean is worthless with its endless ego.' A selfish man always talks about his achievements, and does not have an impressive personality.

It is always good to share. The one who only received his entire life without giving is as good as 'dead'. But the one who never earned much yet donated is a wise man and lives forever. People put money in banks and call it 'dead money' and it is true because it cannot be used to benefit anyone. Wealth is not only gold and silver, but your education which grows when you share it. You should live a life of generosity. A greedy person cannot enjoy his life well. Someone said to the ocean, 'All the rivers come to you and you love them, but you stay away from me.' The ocean replied 'You have created boundaries all around you. First, break all these boundaries and you too can be easily approached and loved by me. I will welcome you here without any greed. When you will be accessible by all, then I will love you more than anyone else.'

Those who are greedy look for their benefit only and never contribute to anything or help others in their entire lives. They are like a well which can never feed others and remain isolated. But those who share receive more from life. The more you donate, the more you shall receive. Those who contribute are considered great. The world's best awards are given for contributions and not for possessions.

Mullah Naseer-ud-din was going somewhere one day when he saw a person drowning in water. People were trying to help him saying, 'Swim to the shore, stay afloat' but he was unable to do so. Then the Mullah approached him and said, 'Take my hand'. The man immediately caught his hand and was saved. The Mullah said 'I offered him a part of me and he was saved.' The one who lives for only himself has no value in life. His life is worthless. One does not get appreciated for earning money but for contributing it. Those who share happiness are great, and succeed.

A king's son was very ill and could not be treated by anyone. A magician appeared and took him to a room. He asked him to burn a paper. As it burnt, the following sentence appeared from the blazing flames - 'Help a person a day'. The child felt happy and was cured.

Aristotle said, 'An ideal person is the one who feels happy on others' successes. The one who feels ashamed to receive help is moving on the path to success. But helping others just to show your strength is foolishness. As flowers do not talk of their fragrance, you too should not show off your qualities. Your qualities should speak for themselves. Try to help others; it will give you peace in life.'

Think before you speak

There was a tortoise living in a pond. There were two birds and they became friends. The birds used to talk about their native country. The tortoise overheard and said, 'Take me to your world. I would like to see that place very much.'

The birds said, 'You cannot fly, so how will you come with us?' The tortoise replied, 'I have a plan. I will latch on to a wooden stick in the middle with my teeth, and the two of you can hold it from either side.' They agreed and started flying. People were amazed to see a tortoise in the air. The proud tortoise shouted loudly, 'Look! I can fly!' As he spoke, his mouth opened, and he fell to the ground and died.

The story tells us that we should be careful about our words and actions. People who talk more have three disadvantages – They talk about meaningless things, they forget whom they are talking to and what the situation is, and they sometimes reveal critical secrets to others due to carelessness. This creates problems for people around them. Hence, think twice before speaking. Rahim has written:

Rahiman jihva bavri, kah gai sarag patar,
Aapan to bhitar gai, jooti khaat kapar.

The tongue is restless and speaks continuously, but creates trouble for the person to whom it belongs. Thus it is very important to control your tongue. Otherwise, it can create hazardous situations for you. One cannot concentrate while speaking, and thus loses efficiency.

A talkative person wastes his entire life talking. His thoughts are shallow and he has no patience. One can focus by being silent, when the mind stops wandering. To be silent means to control your speech and thinking before speaking. Great men say that they succeeded only by controlling their minds and keeping calmness in their hearts. This way, they could reach the highest levels of success. Gandhiji used to practice this habit all the time.

You will also feel a glow on your face and new energy in your body. A talkative person always speaks evil of others and spoils the whole situation. Psychologists say that one can gain energy by being quiet, and also gain greater control over his mind. In this manner, one can concentrate properly and act in the best possible manner according to the situation. Silence can prove to be very strong friend and support in times of crisis.

Two friends in search of a guru approached a saint. They said, 'We are searching for the truth, can you help us?' But the saint remained quiet, so they moved ahead. One of the two boys thought 'How will he teach us when he is mute? Maybe he is quiet to hide his own ignorance – maybe he doesn't know anything'. The other person thought 'He is the real guru – He is proving it with his politeness and calm'. They got separated. Many years later, the second person revisited the guru. He said, 'Gurudev: You taught me the truth that day many years ago by being silent. I am here to thank you.' The saint said, 'Yes, sometimes silence can convey much more powerfully than words.'

It is very important to control your tongue to gain success. Talking more than required can be harmful. A loose tongue can cause anger and fights, thus creating more trouble in life. This small tongue can be responsible for the biggest damages in life and hence must be controlled. We should be very careful while talking, appearing for interviews, speaking in public, etc.

Words are sharper than sword

Swami Vivekananda was explaining about God and one man asked, 'What is the use of words? Why should we learn them?' Vivekananda replied 'You are a fool and an illiterate'. The man got angry and said, 'These words do not suit your character.' Vivekananda replied, 'Did I hit you? So why do you look hurt? My words should have no effect on you.' The man understood the meaning and learned his lesson wisely.

What we say is important. But few people understand this. Most of us cannot control our tongues. We keep on speaking and don't realize when to stop. They want to keep their tongue in motion all the time and speak so much that it is impossible to control them. They repeat the same things over and over, and yet want to speak more about it. They waste all their energy in talking, when they should devote it to constructive work.

Vivekananda's example clarifies that our words can make or break relations and it depends on us. There are many soft spoken people who gently present their words to others. Lal Bahadur Shastri was a very soft spoken person. He was more dedicated inside than his softness outside. His speech contained criticism, anger and humor, yet he was liked by all. Kabir says

Sabad sabad sab koi kahe, sabad ke haath na paun,
Ek sabad aushadhi kare, ek sabad kare ghaav.

One should know the worth of a word and use it wisely. Great men believe that our success and failure depend on our words and it is very important to use them cleverly. People gain best positions in the world by choosing their words wisely. Words have enough power to conquer the entire world, but you need to use it suitably.

Great men think before speaking. Gandhiji had control over his speech always. He was brief and direct in his speech, and remained mute once a week. He said, 'Silence refreshes me.'

Rudyard Kipling said, 'Word can be a powerful medicine.' Therefore, you should be balanced in your speech. Socrates said, 'Your speech is under control till it is not out of your mouth.' Once we have spoken out, it cannot be taken back and we have to live with the consequences.

Therefore, controlling our speech is a key step in the right direction of life.

Thinkers have said that one should think before speaking and make it beneficial for others. We should know when and how to speak, what should be the pace of communication, and what pitch should be used. Those who speak with a proper, underlying theme are always unsuccessful. These people know that speech is an ornament that never fails them in life. In fact, we build our character and stature in society through our speech. It is said;

Bolat hi pehchanie, sahu chor ko ghaat,
Antar ki karni sabai, nikse mukh ki baat.

Yajurveda tells us to speak truthfully at all times. We should give due importance to our words in order to beautify our life and guide it forward in the proper direction. It also beautifies our personality and our place in the society.

Be careful about friends

It is very difficult to find a true friend, but to find a 'phoney' one is very easy – the world is full of 'friends' who are selfish, mean and opportunistic. They will always deceive and hurt you. Beware of the ones who are selfish, competitive, aggressive and unethical. These people have the 'crab mentality' – they are more interested in pulling others down rather than helping them go up. Fortunately, there are many examples of friendship in our history. They inspire us and show us the ideal path of friendship.

What is the true definition of friendship and what does it really mean? Edison said, 'Friendship relieves us from troubles by making us happy.' Ramchandra Shukla said, 'It is like the test of talent of the best doctor, and the patience of a mother.'. Pythagoras said, 'Do not make too many friends as only a few will really come forward to help you in your hour of need.' Confucius said, 'Do not make a friend who is better than you.' This friend will not learn from you and will ignore you. Socrates said, 'Never make friends in haste. It will trouble you in the long run.' Our society is deteriorating and we are at a risk of losing our values in the future. Therefore, the relationships we make today are going to be tested tomorrow, and you have to be ready for it.

Andrew Jackson, the seventh President of United States, shared an interesting experience. His mother wrote to him in a letter, 'Jackson, remember that every human being has to find his own path. For this purpose, he needs friends, so choose them carefully.' Jackson remembered the advice all his life, and never got into trouble.

Our friends play an important role in our success and failure, so they must be chosen very carefully. Everyone struggles for luxuries and comforts of life, but no one cares about true friends. A true friend is an invaluable ally in building a good character. Euripides rightly said, 'There is no better boon to us than a good friend.'

When a friend is so important, why don't we trust him? Has our morals, viewpoints and relations degraded to such an extent? How to find a good friend is a matter of serious concern.

Who should be our friend?

Two friends were travelling through a forest when they saw a bear. The first friend was more concerned with his own safety than that of his friend's, and quickly climbed up a tree, while the second one lay down on the foot of the tree, stopped breathing and pretended to be dead. The bear came, sniffed him and went back. The other boy climbed down and asked, 'What did the bear do?' The other one replied, 'The bear whispered in my ear that a friend who does not help you in trouble is not a true friend and I should beware of such a person.'

There are many people who have 'formal friendships', but stay away during hard times. They are selfish, greedy and clever people. They only say things that you *want* and *like* to hear, and misguide you as per their secret needs and motives. They will run away when you need them the most – we should, therefore, know their real character before we get into trouble.

Know your friends well in schools, colleges, etc. You should help each other in both personal and scholarly life. Every relationship has a 'give and take' factor. But when you ask for help and they say tactfully, 'I am very tired, it is late, I am busy... I can't help you at this moment'. Then you know that this is not a friend worth spending time with. Whether these are your childhood friends, school friends or someone close in the community, you need to take extra care, and make sure you know a person well before offering your friendship. You should never expect any help from them, as they are not going to help you ever in life. Do not be fooled by their sweet tongue; Instead, be charmed by their honest and good intentions towards you.

There is another form of friendship, called companionship. Tulsidas said, *'binu satsang vivek na hoi.'* It means you should stay close to those who teach you valuable lessons in life – this way, you will grow to distinguish about good and evil. It also means that we learn, evolve and grow only in the company of others, not alone. Many a times we are deceived by others, but we have to learn from these experiences too! We need to think how a person is going to affect our life. People who are with you during your happy days are only 'casual acquaintances', but people who are by your side during rough times are your true friends. People who encourage you to indulge in bad habits are not your friends; It is those who show you the right path – despite difficulties – who are true friends worth treasuring.

Therefore, we should be very careful about whom we trust, because our future depends on these relationships. This is the reason our parents stop us from befriending drinkers, smokers and drug addicts. So, we should know the real meaning of friendship and think about it deeply; especially in this day and era where values are disappearing fast, and there are more people to pull us down, rather than pushing us up, the ladder of success.

It's our habit, but...

An addict knows well that drugs, cigarettes, betel leaf, etc. are harmful, but he still continues to consume them. It's a deep seated habit that – in time – becomes very difficult to control. The English thinker Carlyle said, 'It is natural to adopt these habits, simply by indulging in them everyday. Likewise, we can also quit them by trying everyday.'

There was a salesman who used to travel by train on long routes on marketing assignments, which was selling medicines. After retirement, he lost his sleep. He went to the doctor for treatment, but it didn't help. Finally, he found the solution: He bought a bed that was shaped like the berth of a train. From that day, he slept soundly every night.

There are good and bad habits. One has to live with both, and it is natural for us to be habitual.

If we analyze habits, we will find different categories of people. Some become habitual of their professional work, eg, a typist can type without looking at the alphabets, and does so with impressive speed. We all have senses which work by themselves (without active control from our side), and we are habitual of it. There is another type called attitudinal habit. Painters and artists do not see flowers, nature, animals, etc. in the way that we do. It means our thoughts depend on our habits and we create them ourselves. It affects our daily life as it is natural to be surrounded by different habits everyday. A surgeon becomes emotionless while operating because it is his professional habit. A person who works in a slaughterhouse kills animals everyday, but does so without any emotions as this has become his habit.

So, how do we become the victims of habit? Poet John Dryden wrote, 'First we adopt habits once, and then they control us forever.' We begin smoking occasionally, but gradually get addicted to it. Soon, it catches us in a vice-like grip and we then cannot leave this habit ever, and hence end up suffering. On the positive side, we can develop our habits to learn, exercise, boost your mental energy, improve our personalities, etc. Our growth and success purely depend on our habits. Thus, if you want a lucrative future, you must adopt good habits.

The psychologist James said, 'To leave a habit in one go (one sudden jerk) is the best way to get rid of it.' If a smoker tries to cut down his consumption, he can never leave this habit. It should be considered as a poisonous addiction, which has to be controlled completely and therefore has to be destroyed at once, not gradually. It is difficult but one can succeed by showing dedication.

Do not forget that man cannot live without habits. It is a psychological process and is necessary. It will benefit us, therefore, to replace our bad habits with good ones.

Make your habits your servant, not master

Our habits are like twin sisters – bad and ugly, good and beautiful. It is true that good habits take you to success and bad habits take you away from it. These are like steel chains that tie us to them and affect our life greatly – for better or for worse. Bad habits are like landslides that take us down and further down, till our lives are destroyed.

Hence, we should be careful about our bad habits. Instead of becoming their slave, one should strive to become the master because one who is controlled by his or her bad habits can never contribute positively to the society. Those who succeed in life are not the victims of bad habits, but the ones who have learned to conquer and control them. People respect them and they become popular. The growth of good thoughts and habits is rather slow, but consistent, and therefore beneficial to us. We have to learn to complete our tasks in time and that can be accomplished by adopting such a habit.

Thinkers have categorized a habit in four main patterns and aspects. They are as follows:

First is punctuality – to finish all tasks in time, reaching a place on time and knowing its importance, and being considerate of not wasting other's time. The second one is vision – to be careful about bad habits, knowing the difference between good and evil. Third one is dynamism, energy and dedication - you have to continue till the end of the task. A lazy, depressed and effortless person can never progress in life. Those who are dynamic and consistent can succeed in any area and are well respected by all, whereas stagnant people lag behind and no one cares about them. The fourth habit is talent – if we are not talented, then no one will value us and we will lose our importance. It is nice to adopt these habits in life and gain success through them.

Some one has rightly said, 'Human nature has many aspects and our success depends on our character.' Good habits make our lives simple and enriching. It increases our capacity to work, but we must not become careless. Author Ruskin Bond said, 'I feel sorry for those who are careless and for whom it has become a habit.' Man gains bad habits from the wrong company, so we must be very careful about the company you keep. You should try to be with good people all the time. It will help you adopt good habits and help you succeed in life.

Petty is crucial

We generally do not think about petty issues. Gandhiji received a letter with three pages but it was not important. He took out the pin and threw away the letter. The people sitting around asked, 'Why did you throw the letter?' Gandhiji replied, 'I kept what's useful'. Gandhiji used to collect wrappers for his rough work, but never wasted them.

Sometimes, petty issues can be very important in life. Scottish inventor James Watt was waiting near a stove when he saw the water boiling in the kettle. He understood the potential of steam and went on to invent the modern steam engine.

Generally, we do not focus on petty and 'insignificant' things occurring in our life. Our attitude and thinking ability decide our course of action. It can be useful or may be useless. The language that we use is another petty thing that we do not pay much attention to; yet our words are powerful weapons that can hurt others and ultimately ourselves later in life. So, it is better to analyze yourself and control your bad habits in time.

You kept an AK-47 in your house on your friend's request because you never gave it much thought, but it can put you in trouble – the police will arrest you and you will be looked down upon by the society. The court will punish you for what you thought was a 'petty matter.'

Never think that 'small' means 'unimportant'. A small ant can take the life of a huge elephant, a small termite can destroy all the wooden furniture of your house, a mosquito can give you a life-threatening disease. Thus, give importance to all things - whether they seem useless or useful. A needle can do what a sword cannot. It means everything is important to somebody, at some time, in some manner. A small matchstick can create a gigantic forest-fire. Similarly, our little bad habit can, too, blow up and put our life and future in danger.

❑

7

YOUR CHARACTER

- *How is your character?*
- *Examine your character*
- *The mirror never lies*
- *Our language*
- *How to build character?*
- *It happens with politeness*
- *Be humble as you grow*
- *Be a fruit bearing tree*
- *You will reap as you sow*
- *A needle can do what a sword cannot*

How is your character?

Our character is not only the reflection of our qualities but also contains the roots of success. But what is a character? Shouting, showing ego and getting angry is not character. To behave uncouthly, being unethical and speaking without thinking is not character. We have to understand the real meaning of character for which we have to make 'real' efforts in our personal and professional life. Our character is developed on such grounds. This theory is well supported by famous scientists and psychologists.

People with a greater IQ number (IQ = Intelligence Quotient) are considered more intelligent and talented than those with a lower IQ count. Soon, everyone was taking IQ tests to prove and improve their standing and stature in the society. But the concept flopped. It was found that those with greater IQ, while very good at certain areas of life, failed miserably in other areas and subjects. A bookworm may be good in studies, but cannot succeed in many other important domains of life. So what's the use of an IQ score?

Man is intelligent, clever and has many qualities, but is he dedicated to his job? It is necessary to know this because if an intelligent person does not show dedication then what is the use of his intelligence? Thus, we need to know his PQ, or Passion Quotient. Economics guru Arindam Chaudhri says, 'If someone thinks he can do something useful, he should begin it immediately. His steps towards his goal would prove his efforts and passion in life.' Sometimes, we are not dedicated enough and hence do not succeed.

Some people say that Subhash Chandra Bose was unsuccessful because he did not achieve his goal. It may be 'technically accurate' that Netaji didn't achieve his ultimate goal of complete freedom from British rule, it is equally true that Netaji showed legendary courage and bravery. Is the man who has followed his principles and dreams sincerely not successful? These people have a special and different character, and they keep on struggling for their goals. The tougher the challenge, the stronger and more resolved (determined) they become. These people never become irresponsible and are ready to fight any challenge. They seek out challenges, and relish conquering them. They love playing with risks without which they say 'Oh God, what would happen? Please give me more challenges and projects.' Even God helps them, and they accept the challenges. But those who fear their problems achieve nothing in life. You have to work hard, show dedication and believe in God to succeed in life. If you do not follow this path, then you will achieve nothing great in life.

Character is a different dimension altogether, and is clearly apparent in our emotional and spiritual content. We learn to love others from our family, friends, mates and colleagues. We feel glad to meet an Indian in a foreign country and greet them warmly. Gandhiji was the best example of a sound character. Therefore, we must imbibe his qualities and character within us.

Jesus reached a town which was full of cruel, brutal murderers. People gathered to meet Jesus and one asked, 'Could you not find a more peaceful and decent place to visit and stay? Why are you living with these slaughterers?' Jesus replied, 'The doctor visits his unwell patients to treat them... he doesn't visit the healthy ones. So, I am here to treat them.' This is true generosity and we should imbibe this in us. Emerson said, 'A warm and welcoming nature is much more beautiful than a beautiful face. But a sound character is above all. It provides peace, guidance and hope to everyone, which is a rare quality, and a true art.'.

Examine your character

Two singers applied for membership to a music band, and were invited for the auditions in front of a big audience. One of them was weak, upset and did not leave an impact. His song did not 'touch' anyone, while the other candidate was handsome, well dressed and powerfully attracted his audience. As a result, he was selected.

It is necessary to have an impressive personality. It is said 'Character is as necessary for a man as fragrance is for a flower.' Our character is a mixture of our behavior, our routine habits and our inner thoughts. Ego, anger and rude language are not good signs of a character. There are a few qualities that form the foundation of a sound character, and one should adopt these habits. We must respect our elders, especially our parents. We must not boast of our qualities. Many people feel inferior in front of others, and cannot express themselves properly. The reason is that they have no impressive qualities.

One does not need wealth, popularity or achievements to build a sound character; What he needs are self-confidence, self-dependence and ability. We need to develop these habits and apply them in all walks of life. Character cannot be acquired from anyone, not even from ancestors. You can become what you want to be. All you need is to believe in yourself and make efforts. Someone said, 'There is nothing in this world that cannot be achieved. On the other hand, there is no person on this earth who can attain success without affection in his heart and passion in his mind. But with these qualities, he can succeed beyond his wildest imagination.' It has also been said by another thinker, 'Everything is possible for a confident person.'

Those who work with confidence and have passion to achieve their goals nurture their talent carefully, everyday. But the inferior ones lose because they keep crying about their failures and against others' successes. They want to reach the top but fear falling down. One should have dedication and passion in his work to step up the ladder of success. He should not worry about obstacles, and must never be sidetracked from his journey. He should only walk along the path of his aspirations and visions, and leave aside negativity and greed.

Someone who adopts these qualities can never fail in life. We should know our own shortcomings and constantly improve upon them to evolve into a new, positive person. We can eliminate our weaknesses by developing new good habits and thus become capable of receiving and gaining more from life. One cannot succeed until he has eliminated impurity from his mind, since this ruins one's entire image and perspective of life, work and professional goals. Impurities and distractions in the mind can make one careless and irresponsible. Poet Alfred Tennyson said, 'My sword can cut a horse's shoe when it is focussed, and I can dominate ten men because of my pure heart.' Purity is the real power of a person and he can win any battle with it. The person who always follows the truth has success waiting for him. Those who want their character to grow and be successful make an active effort to keep away from bad habits. It is said 'One should protect his character more dearly than his life.'

We need to control our senses and desires to gain a sound character, and it is only possible through sincere self-analysis.

The mirror never lies

Man's character is his true image. When you meet somebody, you easily identify his character in a few minutes. Is he balanced, disturbed or an egotist? Evasive people are easily recognizable and they reflect their personality through their behavior. Behavior is inside us, and we can purify it by expressing our true emotions.

Our character is automatically reflected in our personality. One who suppresses his true feelings can be easily identified – if not today, then definitely tomorrow. People begin to understand him in the long run. One can befool some people every time; one can befool everyone for some of the time, but one cannot befool everyone all of the time. We stop trusting people who are deceitful by nature and they get no respect in the society.

The beauty and secret of life lies in the fact that we should take care of our personality and channelize our potentials in the right directions. This will help us build a strong character and will be helpful in our future. You are the creator of your destiny and no one can help you in this regard. You have to find your weaknesses and eliminate them step by step. A person with a strong character keeps himself active and knows the difference between the different aspects of life. His efforts and self-awareness are his true characteristics.

These traits are not inborn, and have to be acquired by hard work and labour. We can eliminate our shortcomings and develop our character. Once, someone saw Socrates and said, 'This person appears to be lazy and firm.' His friend repeated this observation to Socrates and said, 'I have been your friend for a long time, but am not aware of this aspect of your nature. How could that man say this at first glance?' Socrates said 'He is correct, and has accurately assessed my shortcomings. But it is also true that I have developed my habit.'

A characterless person is always dependent on others and expects everything from them. On the contrary, a man with a strong character believes in his abilities and accepts every challenge with enthusiasm and confidence. He absorbs the best and leaves the rest.

Emerson said, 'A 'real man' will never accept challenges easily, and he will never be impeded by obstacles easily. There is nothing more beautiful or powerful than a pure heart, and the whole world can be yours when you possess these qualities. I taught this to a person who was forcing me to become a Christian. I told him that when it is against my principles, I cannot accept the proposal - I cannot go against my rules and there is nothing better for me than purity in my heart. My duty is not decided by others.'

Remember, character is a lamp that reflects your true personality through your thoughts and actions. Nurturing your character is itself an achievement in life.

Our language

In the epic *Mahabbharata,* Lord Shri Krishna advised Shalya to fight in his favour, said 'You need to discourage Karan'. Shalya asked, 'How can I do this?' Krishna replied, 'When Karan fights, you need to tell him that he is fighting against brave men and cannot win this battle, and that he cannot do anything and will lose this war.' The war began and Shalya did as directed by Krishna. Karan was greatly discouraged and kept fighting a half-hearted war, which eventually claimed his life.

Our speech has more impact on others than our actions, and its effects can be both long lived as well as immediate. You need to think before you speak and control your tongue because it will affect your and others' future. Domestic violence is happening all around us due to bitter words.

The result of sharp and rude language can be easily observed in homes where daughters-in-law are badly beaten, and the story takes the shape of a criminal offense. Drama, crime and violence on television is leaving a bigger and bigger impact on society, and people are fighting in buses, public areas and offices. Every one is using his language like a sword in order to hurt – not soothe – others. We are becoming more and more offensive. If someone talks to us about patience, we sarcastically call him a saint or a lecturer, but don't realize that he is speaking the truth. If we speak evil of others, we will have to face the consequences.

Karan's example clearly showed the impact of words, and it has been scientifically proven too. Why do we forget to think before speaking? We know that we can control animals by loving them – aren't human beings much more evolved than animals? Then why do we create trouble by speaking bitter words and using a harsh tone (instead of employing the even more powerful tools of love, understanding and sympathy)? Everyone has lost control over his language due to ego, jealousy and opposition. We are destroying our society. Vedvyas wrote 'Speech is a weapon that can affect other person deeply and continuously.'

We have to think and practice good speech, and learn the habits of effective speaking. It can solve many of our problems and make our life beautiful. We should not try too hard to be 'ideal', but simply try to be a person with a strong, positive and helpful character. Speaking bitterly can only create trouble. Kabir has said

Madhur vachan hai aushadhi, katu vachan hai teer,
Shravan dwar te sanchare, sale sakal sarir.

So, try to inculcate good speech in your life and you will find tremendous changes in your personality. Others will surely follow you and team up with you to teach more people. Don't depend on TV channels, saints or politicians. Do it yourself. Gandhiji fought the battle of independence. You can too perform this task.

How to build character?

I was reading about Dalai Lama. The Tibetan leader has written, 'You need to know the first step to be happy. We should be aware how our negative thoughts can harm us, or how our positive thoughts can be useful to us. We should also know that negativity is not only harmful to us, but to the whole of society as well.' His words advise us to eliminate negative thoughts from our minds and live with the beauty and harmony of a beautiful life full of positive approach. Our behavior forms the foundation of society, goes on to give shape to our culture, then the nation, and finally, has the power to define and determine the whole world. Hence, it is necessary to develop our emotions and thoughts about life in a positive manner. German philosopher **Friedrich Wilhelm Nietzsche** said, 'A characterless person is harmful to everyone.' So, if we want to develop our character, we should take a giant step and make it a habit in our daily life. You can appear glittering and don the most beautiful clothes and accessories and can drive a luxurious car, but if you lack a sound character then all these aspects can be a waste. Politicians are best examples of it; they wear khadi and show politeness but have been known to be surprisingly 'rough' and 'iniquitous' under the skin. Their fake attitude often reflect in their expressions. They are respected by public, but for how long? Mahatma Gandhi was a simple person and was respected due to his character. Therefore, we should beautify our character.

I want to tell you about Osho who was a person of deep thoughts and had developed his life by controlling his characteristic habits. Osho had said, 'An honest person is not an egoist and is not dependent on society. Society feeds your hungry ego and you enjoy it – gradually, you become dangerously dependent on society. It amplifies your ego but an honest person will see the reality easily. An egotist is deeply involved in himself and hence feels lonely. He tries to fill the gap by gaining physical pleasures and to feel his importance. But truth prevails in the end, and he remains unsuccessful. He is hopeful about his success, but fails on the last step because it is his illusion. At that point, he feels that has no money – it's because he has never heard about the real wealth of life. He never tried to know his inner self.'

We said that people consider physical appearance to be the character of a human being and try to beautify it, but is overwhelmed by sorrow at the end. But by that time, it's usually too late. Osho says, 'People are confused about their internal and external personalities, and misread the situation. Until you leave external traits you will not learn the inner traits of your personality. The more you know yourself, the more you are respected and less dependent you become. The central fact is that you have to grow your inner part and gain more respect than before. But we tend to receive more respect that than offer it. And this leads to harm. What you can gain through physical aspects can also be gained by knowledge. You analyze others and how they feel about you. You show off certain aspects to prove your worth and become social. There are many people who cut themselves off from their inner traits and get busy in outward appearances. So, beautify your inner side first, and the outside world will automatically become glamorous for you.'

Everyone follows this procedure for characterization, but it is important to be passionate about it. If you want real peace in life, then you will have to develop the internal side; but if you want external peace, you will see yourself losing all the great parts and aspects of living.

There is a small anecdote about Osho. People asked the 90-year-old saint, 'You are always happy, what is the secret? You are getting old day by day and you are still happy, what is the reason behind it?' The saint replied, 'There is no secret, but a powerful truth behind it. I learned and decided to choose between heaven and hell. So, when I wake up in the morning I ask myself this question everyday, and my heart wants heaven every time. Thus, I live happily.' It depends on you – what kind of peace you want in life.

It happens with politeness

There was a Shami tree near a river, and a bent tree inside the river. The Shami tree said, 'You are very weak and bend with the waves. Look at me, I am standing straight. Can anyone bend me?' The bent tree said, 'You are great but I believe in politeness.' The Shami tree used to tease the other tree and said 'Only cowards talk like you. There is no one stronger like me.' The bent tree was quiet and did not speak. One day, it started raining heavily and the bent tree stood on its ground even after a flood, but the Shami tree drowned in the water. The bent tree thanked God for his help.

Politeness is our true jewellery, and makes our character shine beautifully. It makes us pure and helps us fight adversities like anger and ego. People do not like to sit with an angry person and they laugh at him. He gets nothing but isolation. On the other hand, the polite and the kind-hearted receive respect and love from everyone. Everyone helps him and wishes for his success.

Charles Dickens was surrounded by people all the time who gathered to learn from him. German writer Goethe was appreciated everywhere he visited. People used to forget their lunch and dinner when he was near. Mirvo was very ugly, but much more respected than beautiful faces. Every cruel person can become polite provided he is kind and considerate to others. Pope Clement XIV greeted some strangers on his appointment and one worker said, 'The Pope should not be humble to his public to such an extent.' But the Pope replied, 'I may have got this prestigious designation, but I cannot forget my politeness and humility.'

The thoughts and behaviors set by our ancestors are steady, firm and significant even in today's world. Our behavior should be polite and humble; it should reflect sweetness and gentleness towards others. We should not treat others how we ourselves would not like to be treated.

Other valuable aspects of our personality are discipline, moral characteristics and social etiquettes. We should be polite and humble while dealing with others. Education is the core and origin of politeness, and it is necessary to be gentle to refine our character. One can improve both physical and social aspects of one's life through education. Hitopdesha says;

Vidya dadati vinayam vinayaati patratam,
Patratvad dhanmanyopoti dhanad tatah sukham.

Education breeds politeness and produces talent. Talent nurtures culture, which brings peace.

There was a fight between holy people and demons, but the holy people were hesitant. They wanted a new commander. Suryavanshi king Raja Muchkund was appointed to lead the holy men. He was very powerful. He defeated many demons and the war continued for a long time. However, the situation changed and they started losing the battle when the king gradually developed an ego and started believing that he was the greatest man on the earth. So another commander Kartikeya was appointed, who advised the king to get rid of his arrogance. The king realized his folly and agreed. He led the holy people to victory.

Saint August said, 'The holy egotist becomes a beast, and polite men become holy.'

Politeness is not only the source of building our character, but also guides the action and thinking of the whole world. Scottish author Samuel Smiles said, 'Politeness has a bigger impact, and it doesn't cost anything, either. It impresses everyone. Sir T Marne said, 'Politeness is respect to seniors, duty to mates, love to juniors and protection and guidance to society.' A polite person is acknowledged as great. Kabir said;

Sabte laghutai bhali, laghuta te ab hoye,
Jis dwitya ko chandrama, sheesh navai sab koi.

We need to remember that one should not have an ego of being polite. Marcus rightly said, 'There can be nothing worse than being an egotist for your politeness.' Wordsworth said, 'When we bow down, we are closer to intelligence.' An intelligent mind is recognized by his politeness. Founder of Pennsylvania William Penn said, 'Intelligence multiplies with politeness. It is a precious jewel of character.'

Gandhiji used to perform all his domestic tasks in Sabarmati Ashram himself – tasks that were generally done by servants. Vinobha Bhave used to draw water from the well in his ashram, without help from anyone.

We too should be polite because it improves our character.

Be humble as you grow

Lal Bahadur Shastri was a very humble and jovial person. When he was a Member of Parliament, he did not want his name to be printed in the newspapers. One of his friends asked the reason and Shastri replied, 'Lala Lajpat Rai once told me that there are two types of marbles in the Taj Mahal. One is sangmarmar which is appreciated by all and shines all the time. The other is in its foundation on which it stands, and cannot be seen.' It's easy to guess the qualities of a person who follows this principle.

Politeness is the key to gain respect and appreciation. We might have a huge fan following, but the kind of outlook and character we adopt in life depends on us. It is said that a high thinker is admired by all. He has no ego in him. Gandhiji said that politeness means the elimination of ego.

It was ego that led to the Second World War and the evil designs of the Nazis to dominate the world. It was the cause of the massacre that happened in Hiroshima and Nagasaki. Politeness leaves when ego enters and you stop progressing. Your ego will create obstacles in your path and no one will offer you help. People will say, 'He is an egotist and cruel.' You will feel hurt, lonely and miserable, and it will lead to disaster. Be polite and follow the 'Live and let live' slogan.

Tulsidas has written that a polite person does not contain any faults. Nature wise, he remains static in all situations. He is happy with what he receives and never feels jealous. An egotist, on the other hand, feels jealous about those superior to him. He is always greedy and wants to imitate others. Rabindra Nath Tagore said, 'We are closer to greatness when we are polite.'

Lord Buddha, Jesus and Gandhi adopted politeness in their personal lives, and taught us to love everyone. Jesus said, 'If someone slaps you, show him the other cheek.' Gandhiji said, 'A person without a polite nature cannot utilize his potential.'

Indian author Ruskin Bond rightly said, 'I believe that the mark of a gentleman is his politeness.'

When we are polite, everybody loves talking to us. On the other hand, impolite people are criticized and avoided by everyone. It is said that politeness has no room for partiality and treats every one equally. Therefore, we should be polite. We can gain respect at home, at work and in society by being polite. If you do not believe this theory, try it yourself.

Be a fruit bearing tree

A tree is a beautiful example of politeness. They bend down when they bear fruit so that we may eat the fruits. It does not have any ego. Trees underline the importance of politeness in our life. People respect polite people, treat them with politeness in return, and listen attentively to their words. But egotists are not liked by anyone, and are avoided by all.

There was a king who decided to donate money everyday. He became popular and built a charity house with forty doors. He used to donate money to everyone and announced it publicly. One day, a beggar arrived in his kingdom and the king gave him a gold coin. He stood at the next door and the king again gave him some money. When he reached the third door, the beggar got some more money. At every door, he collected a gold coin. When he reached the fortieth door, the king asked, 'Are you not satisfied?' The beggar replied, 'I wanted to test your patience and politeness. You have much ego inside. You are telling me that you donate money. Who are you to donate? God does this charity, you are only the medium.' The beggar returned the gold coins and went back. The king learnt his lesson and was ashamed of his behavior.

One who is not polite and has no ethics has no value in society. If you consider seriously, you will understand that ethics and politeness are two sides of the same coin. People with these qualities are considered great, and it is necessary for all of us to apply it in our lives. You cannot be polite in the presence of ego.

We have forgotten the importance of politeness and ethics in our society. A polite person is criticized and befooled by others. How can we change this trend? Would you like to gift these habits to the next generation? We have to build a new era of truth and politeness. We have to nurture our potential and fight against unethical behavior. We have to reprimand the foul-mouthed person and learn to raise our voice against rude mannerisms. Not speaking against crime is a bigger crime. We have to oppose the unethical behavior of the society we live in.

It is easy to understand the value of politeness and ethics for the progress of a human being. We cannot reject our traditional values as they play an important part of our personality. Confucius said, 'Politeness is the basis of good qualities – even nature teaches us the same. Water flows smoothly and takes the shape of the vessel it is poured into.'

Kalidas said,

Bhavanti namratshav falod garmanin
vambhubhibhuri vilimbano Ghana,
Anudhtta satya puruhshibhi samridhibhi
swabhav avaish paropkarinam.

The tree bends on bearing fruits, clouds do the same when it rains, educated souls become more polite on earning wealth. This is the mark of a true gentleman. People consider politeness and ethics to be weaknesses, but they couldn't be more wrong. These are the characteristics of an intelligent mind. We have to set an example and then we can teach others to follow it.

You will reap as you sow

Ethical behavior makes our personality beautiful. One with ethical behavior is always admired and he respects others as well. Western poet Edison said, 'Politeness is the bridge to the inner soul.' A proverb says, 'We reap what we sow'. We are rewarded for our good deeds and we have to pay for our evil tasks. One who thinks about it seriously never uses slang. He thinks good of others and is loved by all. Abraham Lincoln was criticized by many, but he was polite and humble towards everyone. He went on to become the President of USA, the most powerful country in the world. Lincoln never fired any deserving person from a post, even though he was criticized by the latter. He thanked God, but did not respond to his critics. He, instead of taking action, used to pray for his opponents. Never waste your time in thinking about your rivals. These thoughts provoke poor qualities and hence we must stay away from them.

One must be humble and polite to all, and should not treat others in an improper manner. One is known by these qualities and loved because of them. The more humble a person is, the more he will be polite to others. Somebody asked Lukman, 'From where did you learn this habit of politeness?' He replied, 'From unethical people. I used to observe their behaviour carefully, and make my best effort not to follow them!'

It is worthwhile to remember that one should not expect the same behavior from others as we treat them. We cannot hope for civilized behaviour from others – they may, or may not, be courteous to you. Jesus cured ten patients and only one thanked him – he was Saint Luke. Expecting from others leads to disappointment. Aristotle said, 'An ideal man is one who feels peace in helping others but is ashamed about taking others' help.' Accepting good habits is not an inferior thing; it involves a good character, dedication and culture. You should not speak poorly about others even though he does not love you (and, in fact, loathes you). We should develop this habit and learn from other's mistakes.

Thus, we should imbibe only those habits that develop our character. It will nurture our heart and thoughts, and make our life beautiful.

A needle can do what a sword cannot

As Rabindranath Tagore steadily gained popularity for his literary works, some people began to envy him. They started writing wrong information about him in the newspapers to smear his image. But he was not affected by it and did not react to them. Sharatchandra Chatterjee didn't like this and asked him, 'Why do you not respond to the critics?' Tagore replied, 'They have adopted wrong means and are harmless to me. My politeness is my answer to them.'

Politeness can do what a war cannot. It wins hearts while the latter can win only a battle – but at the cost of many lives. There are many situations where we have to prove ourselves and these are the times of our personality test. The best way is to be polite. It is not good to respond sharply, as this only provokes anger. Our mentors, planners and saints teach us the same values and ethics. We should be polite by nature and not harm others. According to Buddhists, 'Shishta khul vigatamtsara nirhankara kumbhi dhanya alolupa dambhandarpalobhmah krodhvivarjita', i.e., one who is not jealous, egotist, greedy or angry is called an ethical person.

It is the quality of a person that reflects in our personality. Our moral values should be our politeness and humbleness. The one who respects others is an ethical person. Bhass said, 'Polite people never get angry.' A saint heard that one can eliminate anger by praying to God, and he went to the Himalayas for the same. When he returned, many visitors came to meet him and he considered himself a great personality. He had an inflated ego and scolded a disciple who was massaging him. He said, 'Don't you know me, I am a great saint.' The person felt hurt and said, 'Is he a saint? He is a fool and has no ethics. How will he preach others?' The saint heard this and was ashamed. His prayers in the Himalayas had gone to the waste.

Poet Kalidas said, 'Politeness is the most attractive part of humanity.' Politeness can be applied and experienced in different ways in different cultures, but, at its core, is one and the same concept everyone. It teaches us the values of life and protects us from evil. It is based on giving respect to others and receiving the same.

A thinker said, 'Ethics is a combination of many qualities as it is a culture and a behaviour. One cannot be uncouth and unethical. The one who is blessed with its fragrance can never speak ill words. He is peaceful and behaves in the same way to others. This quality rises from deep, inner values, and brings joy and success in life.'

Lilli Allen also said in this context, 'Ethical people are not flashy, and behave in a balanced manner in every situation.' Emerson said, 'An ethical man never shouts and an ethical woman always speaks softly. We should take care of our behavior and nurture it. Those who know the path of politeness attain happiness. He is able to take care of his behavior in every situation. One cannot sacrifice great qualities at any cost.'

A saint was going through a town with his students when somebody threw ash on them. The saint thanked them and his student asked, 'Why did you thank them?' The saint replied, 'God is favorable to us. If he had thrown fire, we could have burned. We are safe now, so I thanked them.'

Ethical people never shout and find positive things in life. Those who are uncouth fight with others and make blunders. Mistakes do not happen intentionally, and should be ignored with consideration and kindness. When one throws a stone in the mud, one gets dirty himself. Thus, we should be careful about our behavior and control it at all times. We should not forget the words of great thinkers, 'Our politeness and respect depends on our behavior.' Angry people, unsatisfied men and jealous people never feel healthy or peaceful in their minds, and react accordingly. They first harm themselves and then others. At the end, they meet failure and get insulted. Dissatisfied people have many obstacles in their path that drag them to failure. They develop many enemies and discourage everyone.

We should practice being polite and humble. It will benefit us by winning laurels and smoothening the flow of success.

❑

8

ANXIETY & WORRY

- *Anxiety can lead to downfall*
- *Stay away from anxiety*
- *Why are we doubtful?*
- *What is the result of stepping on it?*
- *Unusual demands*
- *Slow and steady wins the race*
- *If you chase two rabbits simultaneously, both will escape*
- *Yes, you can*

Anxiety can lead to downfall

We often feel tensed in our everyday life. Businessmen worry about their business, employees are worried about their jobs, an apprentice is worried about his selection, and the patient is worried about his health.

The truth is that worry is an important and inseparable part of life and makes us knotty and hollow from the inside. Anxiety leads us to the end.

There are several reasons for anxiety – but all of them can be solved simply by being happy. Being successful or not is one of the reasons. We are scared of failing in exams, competitions and in other areas of life, and we worry about it. We are struck between success and failure. This is totally useless and creates frustration that leads to failure. No one can help us, but ourselves. We have to solve the problem ourselves and need not fear.

Psychologists say that anxiety leads to physiological imbalance and results in disease and illness. A person becomes a heart patient or a victim of other fatal diseases, and starts suffering in his personal life. We are ruining our health by worrying for no reason. 'I should become successful so that people respect me, and I must earn wealth' – these are the main reasons for anxiety and one should be careful about them.

These demands are useless and hence we need to remain away from anxiety. We should not worry because, in either case, we do not know if our wishes will come true or not. Therefore, we should remember that worry creates more worry and ultimately destroys us. We become incapable in our work and in our lives, and go down in every sense. We should never worry at all, and practice courage, bravery and intelligence in our life.

Stay away from anxiety

French guru Mariyek said, 'When someone asks me in this virtual world about my belief in God, I reply – He relieves me from my anxiety.' Worry surrounds us from childhood – we fear from darkness. We worry in school life about education and exams. What is the use? Will our worry answer the questions in our mind? No.

We have many reasons to worry in life, but no reason to smile. When we do someone a favor, we start expecting love, affection and help in return. We are worried about our jobs, children, their education and health, and the family's well being. We are fully surrounded by anxiety in every aspect in our lives. We are worried about finding solutions to our worries. It is rightly said, 'Worry is like a honey bee - it will stick as you try to remove it.'

We are always busy worrying about our future. Thinkers say, 'We should not worry about the future as nothing will happen according to our wishes. If we have to worry, we should worry for success.'

Beecher said, 'One does not die from work, but from worrying about it.' One remains healthy by working, but worrying destroys us – just like rust destroys a blade. A machine doesn't deteriorate when worked upon, but gradually disintegrates if left idle. It is regrettable that most of us surrender to worries and tension. We do not find peace in life and always remain scared. We should move towards our goals with prior planning and confidence.

A person lost one eye and began to worry about his future. He lost sleep and his other eye also developed the same problem. He consulted a doctor who advised him to take rest. And he recovered quickly. Our worries are not going to help our future constructively… it can only spoil it. Thus, we do not dare take risks and lag behind in life.

We are surrounded by materialistic opportunities and we worry about them. We are demanding more from life everyday, and lose our inner peace in the process. We are never satisfied and feel jealous about others. Weak students worry during exam time and forget the answers in the exam hall. Thinkers say, 'The easiest solution is to forget worrying and start working.' Never regret in life for what has already happened and do not worry about what is not going to happen. You can push away your anxiety with your internal power. Do not waste your time and do some creative task instead. One can gain peace by being happy.

Former British Prime Minister Winston Churchill worked 18 hours a day during World War II. Somebody asked him, 'You have many problems, yet you are not worried.' He replied, 'I don't have the time to worry.'

George Bernard Shaw said, 'To think of trouble when the mind is relaxing is the real cause of our troubles. If you have a leisure period, do something constructive - never sit idle. It will guide your mind correctly, and you will find peace in life.' We should utilize each and every moment of our time and enjoy it with others. We are worried about what is not going to happen to us, and fall ill. A writer writes 'If a ship could think, then it would have started to worry about the waves in the ocean that could sink it, and it would have never be able to sail across the seas 'in peace'. Most of our worries are useless and futile. Those who worry about their future ruin their present, and put their future in danger. They are people who do not believe strongly in themselves, or in God. They can never become great.

We are so worried about planning our tasks that we remain doubtful about executing them and as a result do not initiate it. We tie ourselves with the chains of anxiety and lose all our potential. All our efforts become weak and it results in – what we had worried about – failure.

Be calm and stop worrying about worthless objects. Begin your task with confidence and accomplish it. You will succeed if you step up with confidence. Never worry about the problems until you see them. Be creative in your job and never stray in your thoughts. A person asked a donkey, 'What does life mean to you?' The donkey replied 'To graze on grass that is fresh and green.' Then the man asked a buffalo the same question and it replied, 'To enjoy life in the water.' Then he asked a laborer the same question and he shouted back, 'Do you not have any work? Why are you so worried about life? Make it useful and let me do my own work.' We need to make our life useful and beautiful, and stop worrying.

Why are we doubtful?

One has to face competition in every field of life – be it education, job, business, sports, science, history, etc. As a result, people are in a constant state of tension. The number of diseases like heart disease, diabetes, etc. have increased a hundredfold and, unfortunately, has become a part of our life. We ourselves are the creator of the tensions and troubles in our lives and only we can eradicate it. The main reason of stress is fear and we fear from failing in exams, competitions, interviews, business, etc.

Vivekananda used to say, 'Fear creates trouble and is the main cause of stress and failure.' Thus, we should gain control over our fear and the root cause of stress will be eliminated. Gandhiji said, 'The one serving humanity does not fear from anyone but God.' Tensed people are always in trouble and surrounded by a hundred and one diseases. Even medicines cannot cure us sometimes.

Thinkers have said that we should destroy our fear to remove stress from our life. One should know the reasons of fear and try to solve them. Confidence can help us achieve this goal. A person's confidence, self-reliance and dedication are so strong that they can uproot the cause of anxiety and overcome any obstacle. It is said that our fears are unreal and imaginary, and we invite even more anxiety by consulting astrologers. What is the solution? Do not have illusory and cloudy thoughts in your mind. Until you appear in an exam, how will you fail? Prepare well and you will succeed. Intelligent people are aware of their potential and use it wisely. It is not difficult to cross a river if you know how to swim.

First, you have to be committed to the task and train your will-power in order to control your stress. You can destroy your fear as this is created by your own self. A tensed person quits his task mid-way, but if one has a strong will-power, then nobody can stop him from succeeding. Whenever you feel tensed, take a deep breath and forget the cause of your fears. Calm yourself. There is not a single problem in this world which does not have a solution. So think about practical ways to solve your problems because the solution *is* out there; you just have to find it. This will add to your confidence and you will find true happiness inside, along with the solution to your problems. Just try it once and you will feel calm and confident.

Will our worrying about *any* thing help *any* one in *any* way? Instead, we should put our maximum efforts in developing our confidence. Talk to yourself and say, 'I am capable, I can achieve my goals.' Work for it and success will be yours. Sometimes, you can remove your fear by sharing it with your friends, and they will increase your confidence and encourage you to succeed.

Some people smoke or drink in order to get relief from stress. But it is only an illusion that drugs relieve stress. These habits only make us more weak. We feel more stressed and lose confidence, and we fail in every walk of life. Thus, be peaceful and enjoy each moment of life. You can easily control the causes of fear with confidence. A confident person never feels tensed and moves ahead with concentration and achieves his goals.

What is the result of stepping on it?

We want to live a peaceful life and consult gurus for the same, but we do not achieve it. Every one wants to be peaceful, but worries more about it than in trying to actually achieve it. They want instant answers and million-dollar-solutions, but do not check the validity and practicality of their wishes and demands.

A thinker has said, 'The reason behind our worry is the erosion of our values. We are being emptied of our intelligence and drained of our inner potential.' Man is entrapped in this maya of ambitions, wants and the pressures of success, and fake gurus are taking advantage of this. We are stressed by materialistic things and we have lost control of ourselves. We do not make efforts in succeeding but degrade others instead. We worry for no reason and ultimately, our health and our family pay for our mistakes.

People are worried about their success and failure, and as a result they become feeble because they let their worries dominate them. There are people who fear from everything and fail to succeed. Our thoughts have immense effect on our actions. A thinker said that each of our thought creates an action and when someone talks about fear with you, it also amplifies those negative senses in your body. It has been proven that emotions have an effect on man's efficiency. If the mind is peaceful, a person can recuperate from any disease. On the other hand, a doctor will have to make an extra efforts to cure a patient who is stressed and feeble. Dr. William S Edler said, 'The scientific effects of the mind on the body – that our rishis of ancient time used to know very well – have recently been proved. A healthy person can be encountered by disease and a patient can also think for his good health.'

Thus, worrying about a problem and fearing from it is foolishness. The more we fear, the more it scares us. We will be in trouble and lose our potential. As a result, we will be pushed to the edge of failure.

The best ways to bounce back from stress is to think creatively and forget about problems. A famous thinker said, 'A person does not die from work but because of worrying about it.' Work makes one healthy, but worry is like rust on blade. So, be happy at every moment of life, and you will have superior health.

A lady told her husband, 'We have to pay the rent on the sixth of this month.' The man said, 'Then do not worry for the next five days. There is no stipulation of worrying in our Rent Contract.' We forget that we cannot solve the problem by worrying about it. But it is true that we never detach ourselves from worrying about the future. It makes our life complex rather than simplifying it, because we lose our intelligence by worrying.

Shakespeare said, 'I believe anxiety to be an enemy of human beings.' Those who worry feel tensed and ruin their health. Ultimately, worrying and diseases finish them.

A saint said, 'I never worry in life because I know that I will be able to complete my job.' Anxiety is a disease that has a negative effect on our body. According to psychologists, the more we get angry, the more we feel tensed and invite many diseases, thereby losing our health. Doctors have proven the effect of thoughts on the body. If one is peaceful, he can recuperate quickly, but a healthy person can invite many diseases just by worrying. In reality, a person continuously puts thoughts in his subconscious mind and the mind starts working according to the orders directed to it.

Therefore, what is the answer? The solution is that we should focus on the real task-at-hand, and try to solve the problem rather than worrying about it. If you worry, your mind will be surrounded by fear and depression will attack you. This will compel you to lose your thinking and working ability. Thus, think for a solution, be peaceful and concentrate. You will definitely find relief from your pain.

Unusual demands

The worst curse in today's life is stress and every person is tensed with some reason or other. Everyone is running after money-related problems. In the office, business, job, education, etc., there is no calm person. This anxiety is causing fear and is the main generator of diseases. It has reached villages too, in the form of envy, debts, agricultural problems, etc. Although invisible initially, gradually it brings down one's health, and it deteriorates very badly in the later stages. Most of us are suffering from heart disease, headache, diabetes, etc. Worry is the creator of all these diseases and has scattered its many arms to cause trouble in various aspects of our life.

What is stress? It is a toxic substance that takes us towards disaster and makes our minds and lives hollow. It was observed at the time of the Second World War where it imbalanced and unsettled even the best of minds and caused worldwide destruction. American psychologists Thomas Holmes and Richard Rode researched on this topic and uncovered many myths and facts on this problem.

We said that stress has grown due to the rat-race to gain materialistic possessions and it is a world where we can make it to the top only by creating a competitive world around us. Failure creates stress in our mind and we adopt more bad habits like jealousy, doubt, fear, etc. Fear and anxiety arise from suppressing emotions and jealousy. This fear of 'The unknown' causes strain in our mind and we are hounded by diseases.

People who are mean are worried about their doubts and try to hide it from others. This creates more stress as they have to worry about hiding the truth. Is there any solution to this problem? No, no one can cure it but us. If we want, we can even cure it without any medicine and aid. Those who have no faith in reality are tensed in life and imagine unknown fears. This attitude has to be changed and positive thoughts need to be adopted by us.

The only solution to escape from these problems is to stop thinking about it. Concentrate on some other useful activity for a period of time and when you feel relaxed, execute your plans as per your decision. One should not worry about petty issues and say, 'I do not fear from them, these cannot affect me' and you can win your challenges. Psychologists say that a confident person is least affected by fear, and gurus say that the best way to fight fear is to believe in God and his abilities. A firm believer is always aided by God in relieving stress.

Thus, we need to become self-confident and strive to control our thoughts. Never give up showing courage - otherwise, your anxiety will start getting the better of you.

Slow and steady wins the race

People are so worried in their hectic life schedules that they cannot focus on themselves. Statistics tells us that 4.5 crore people are under stress and 25% of world's population is affected by one kind of illness or other. They might not be physically handicapped, but they are mentally handicapped because of their worries and high levels of stress. This is akin to inviting diseases and fueling our inner fears. One cannot be in danger if he is physically hurt, but is in a fatal situation when he is mentally distressed.

In India, you will find many stressed people in search of peace, but not finding it. If we make an effort, then we can definitely protect ourselves from worry without spending a penny. The results can be positive if you are ready to practice it.

What is the root cause of mental problems? It is a stressed mind. The stress in our mind depends on the load of work we have and our attitude towards it. Thus, we have to learn the following 'One has to have healthy mind for a healthy body.' It is believed that when the mind is in peace, it keeps the body healthy; else it becomes the reason for failure. For example, fear forces us to take up a rough and offensive posture in life and society, where we are always mentally ready for a fight. But once we relax both in body and mind, we will feel calm, composed and peaceful inside.

The Bhagwad Gita says 'One who has no desires can have a peaceful life as desires create stress in our mind.' People want to earn more day by day and are worried about it. They are running after success but in the opposite direction and will achieve nothing in life. As you control your demands, you too can feel relaxed and attain a state of peace. It lies inside you and no one can get it for you.

The easiest way to relieve stress is to sit quietly and relax your body. Spiritual guru Dada Vaswani said, 'When you sit quietly, you get energized and it calms your mind. Then, you experience miracles and attain peace forever.' Thus, be quiet as it brings peace in life.

It is very important to control your thoughts in this hectic life; otherwise, it will result in accidents and diseases. In recent times, there has been a marked increase in the number of such patients in the world, with many of them taking up drugs to get relief from stress. But this acts like fuel in fire. Hence, we should deeply think about it as our future depends on it.

Some people show passion and want to grow ahead of others very fast, and as a result find themselves under stress. Once that happens, their performance graph goes down day by day. They become alert to attain peace, but this increases only their anxiety, and they get trapped inside a vicious cycle.

Heed the warning signals well in time and take precautionary action.

Sometimes, people struck in everyday problems do not get time to solve such problems. But the true reason behind your stress is your attitude towards it. You are right, but you have to find a solution for this and attack the roots of your problem. Try it and you will observe positive changes in life.

Osho says, 'There is nothing called a 'problem'. If you still want to absorb it and be affected, it is your wish. Enjoy it and I bless you. But life is a secret which is unknown and has to be followed by us. You create your own problems and then fear them.' You say, 'How can I enjoy my life? I have many problems in life,' or you say 'How can I love my spouse? I have no time to think about him or her. Should I think of my problems or enjoy the music?' It means you are always surrounded by problems created by you and stop yourself from enjoying life. You become a slave of your problems and act upon its orders. If you think deeply, you will find that these problems are imaginary. If you think that these problems are real, even then they can be solved by saying 'Ok, but these can be destroyed. Until I fight courageously, I cannot overcome problems. Hence, I need to focus on my attitude to solve these problems. If I accept the truth and work at it, my life will be peaceful.'

If you chase two rabbits simultaneously, both will escape

The reasons of stress could be many. Since there is no end of desires, there is no satisfaction in life. But we tend to forget that worrying about anything creates trouble in our life and makes it full of disasters. If we want to live, we have to be simple and peaceful. It helps to learn and discover more about great men who have learnt to live with peace in their minds, and pick up valuable lessons from their lives.

A writer was always worried about something or the other – job, health, family, etc. He wasted 10 precious years of his life and could not relish the taste of his age from 18 to 28. He felt inferior inside and stopped meeting people. He used to change his path when any known person approached him and avoided people as much as possible. He could not face strangers and as a result lost his confidence. He could not say, 'I can do this' as he was doubtful of his capabilities. As a result, he lost three job offers. He met a friend after a few years, and he found him smiling in the hard times. He asked his friend, 'How can you smile in this situation?' His friend replied, 'I earned a lot of money through hard work and lost all in one moment. Then, I earned money for four years again and lost it too. I was bankrupt and under a heavy debt. Anyone could have committed suicide in those circumstances, but I bore all those problems and overcame them with my efforts.' He showed a letter full of threatening words and the writer asked, 'How did you reply this letter?' He replied 'It will be solved by keeping the letter closed. It relieves me from mental pain, and I feel I should be calm and patient, during difficult time. The writer applied this formula and learned the art of living and learning peacefully. He understood that every problem is healed with time.

Sir William Osler's book is truly inspiring. He was not only a great doctor but a great human being as well, and his thoughts always help one to relieve one's tension. Once, while receiving an award, he said, 'The credit of all my success goes to the power that helped me make efforts to reach this position, and I make it responsible for my future as well.'

A parrot was sitting in a verandah and kept saying to passers-by *'Ekahi sadhe sab sadhe, sab sadhe sab jaye.'* It means that if you want to succeed, you need to concentrate on a single particular task with all your efforts and commitment. This is the secret of success and the art of living.

❑

Diamond Books Presents

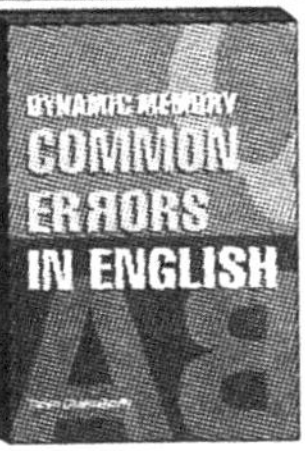

Dynamic Memory Common Errors in English

Tarun Chakarbory

English is a widely used language in our business & professional environment and further in corporate world it is a must. It may be very closely observed that for most of the times, the English used by people is not correct, yet it is spoken and written out of ignorence in the same way. Such show is rated as very bad by learned people. This book by Tarun Chakraborty is a result of his great efforts where he has identified such common errors and presented their correct use. **Rs. 110.00**

Dynamic Memory Perfect Spoken in English

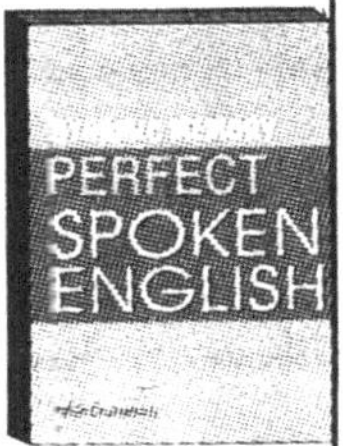

Tarun Chakarbory

English speaking is generally latest as a impressive tool among all class of people. But for most of the times the spoken English is not correct rather it is full of errors. At a glance, such incorrect spoken English is marked behind fluency but it is categoried as a poor show by learned people. This valuable book of Tarun Chakarborty is a meaning full effort to catch the attention of people to correct themselves. The book provides a lot of material to meet the objective. **Rs. 110.00**

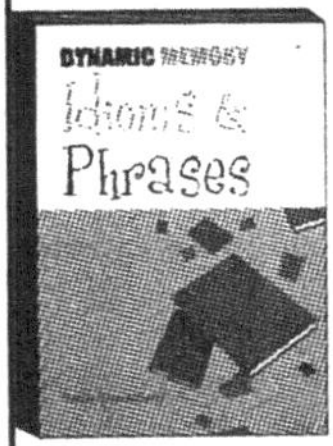

Dynamic Memory Idioms & Phrases

Tarun Chakarbory

This book 'Dynamic Memory Idioms & Phrases' is well written by Sri Tarun Chakraborty to offer a huge collection of idioms, with this idiomatic origin and further their meaning. The idioms are arranged in alphabatic order which is of great help to book user 'the help is further supplemented by content index given at the begin of the book. The book is certainly very valuable for student & English lovers. **Rs. 95.00**

Dynamic Memory Group Discussions

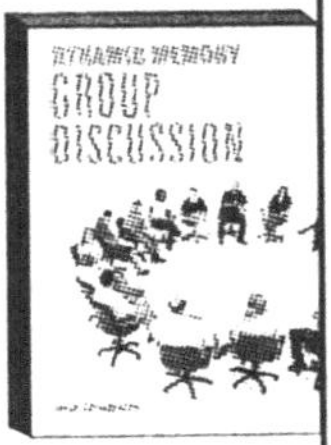

Tarun Chakarbory

Group discussion is a very effective tool to select propes manpower for any good jobs. A candidate has to project his skills of expression to the board, at the same times has to slow that he is good to work in a team, while he is a brilliant leader like person as well. It is a tought experience to overcome group discussion if one is not practical & orient for such game. This book by Tarun Chakarborty steps to precse up this gap and tends to remove the obvious hitch in the candidates. Rs. : **95.00**

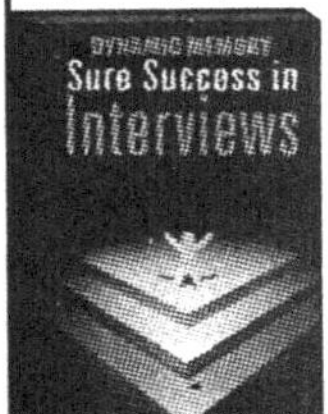

Dynamic Memory Sure Success in Interview

Tarun Chakarbory

When you are invited to an interview it means that the hiring manager believes you may be a good match for the job opening, she or he want to know for sure. This book is a ready reckoner for those who want to present themselves in a powerful & prossive way.

Rs. : 95.00

Dynamic Memory Synoniums & Antonimous Dictionary

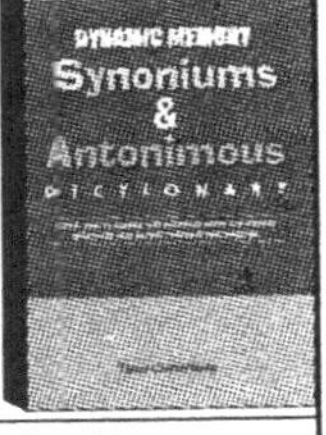

Tarun Chakarbory

Communication is effective when we have a firm grip on vocabulary. Anyone should make the reader's job easier by communicating whatever he or she wants to communicate.

Not only does reading allow you to build up your vocabulary, but it also allows you to become more informed, learning things about the world around you. **Rs. : 95.00**

Books can be requisitioned by V.P.P. Postage charges will be Rs. 20/- per book.
For orders of three books the postage will be free.

DIAMOND BOOKS

X-30, Okhla Industrial Area, Phase-II, New Delhi-110020,
Phone : 41611861 Fax : 41611866
E-mail : sales@dpb.in Website : www.dpb.in